Delivering Quality Diabetes Care in General Practice

Dr Roger Gadsby

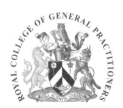

ROYAL COLLEGE OF GENERAL PRACTITIONERS

The Royal College of General Practitioners was founded in 1952 with this object:

"To encourage, foster and maintain the highest possible standards in general practice and for that purpose to take or join with others in taking steps consistent with the charitable nature of that object which may assist towards the same."

Among its responsibilities under its Royal Charter the College is entitled to:

"Diffuse information on all matters affecting general practice and issue such publications as may assist the object of the College."

British Library Cataloguing-in-Publication Data
A catalogue record for this book is available from the British Library

© Royal College of General Practitioners, 2005
Published by the Royal College of General Practitioners 2005
14 Princes Gate
Hyde Park
London
SW7 1PU

Disclaimer
This publication is intended for the use of medical practitioners in the UK and not for patients. The authors, editors and publishers have taken care to ensure that the information contained in this book is correct to the best of their knowledge, at the time of publication. Whilst efforts have been made to ensure the accuracy of the information presented, particularly that related to the prescription of drugs, the authors, editors and Publisher cannot accept liability for information that is subsequently shown to be wrong. Readers are advised to check that the information, especially that related to drug usage, complies with information contained in the *British National Formulary*, or equivalent, or manufacturers' datasheets, and that it complies with the latest legislation and standards of practice.

Designed and typeset by Discript Limited
Printed by Latimer Trend & Co Ltd

ISBN: 0 85084 296 4

*To my wife Pam, and children Emma and Andrew,
for their love and support*

FOREWORD

I am sure that I am not the only general practitioner who feels thoroughly confused by diabetes. I know how incredibly important this condition is. I know that the demographic projections for its incidence are horrifying, with the number of people with diabetes worldwide set to double over the 13 years to 2010. I know that high quality medical care is vitally important, that all diabetic patients should have a general practitioner, and that most diabetic care is carried out in primary care. However, as general practice has become inevitably more specialised, I also know that my own personal knowledge and understanding of the condition has progressively atrophied. When I diagnose diabetes, I ask Martin (one of my partners) to take over the care of this condition in my patient. His care is exemplary; mine would be amateur. I know which my patients deserve.

But I still need to understand this condition. I need to understand current views on therapy, diagnosis, and treatment. I need to deal with the multiple co-morbidities, which mean that diabetes is inevitably a condition that needs a generalist perspective, and I need to be able to answer the questions that my patients continue to ask.

Roger Gadsby's book comes as a breath of fresh air. Taking a genuine general practice perspective, this book recognises the importance of offering high quality care to our patients, and explicitly links this to the targets and points in the new GMS contract. It features case histories of real patients, a table of relevant Read codes, and expertly blends together all the guidelines and studies that have come our way over the past few years – from the NSF to NICE guidelines and all stations in between. Reading this book has answered one of the main educational needs in my own personal development plan, but much more importantly, it will improve the care that I can offer my patients.

If you are your practice's expert on diabetes, or practice in a small practice where you have no choice but to develop the expertise, then this book will be an invaluable digest of information. If like me, you struggle with keeping up to date in this complex condition, this book will provide almost everything that you need.

General practice is the hardest medical speciality to do well. This book wonderfully illuminates the care of this complex, common, and crucial condition. General practitioners, and their patients, will be genuinely grateful that Roger Gadsby has written it. I certainly am.

David Haslam, CBE
Former Chairman of Council,
Royal College of General Practitioners.

CONTENTS

BIOGRAPHY

Dr Roger Gadsby qualified in medicine from Birmingham University in 1974. After postgraduate training he joined the Redroofs practice in Nuneaton in 1979, and is now senior partner of this eight-doctor teaching practice.

He began a practice diabetes clinic in 1984 and has been speaking and writing about diabetes ever since, with over 100 published articles and papers. He was a founder member of PCD UK, the primary care section of Diabetes UK, and has served on a number of national diabetes working groups.

Since 1992 he has been working part-time as a senior lecturer in primary care at Warwick University where he has helped to develop diabetes education programmes. He is medical advisor to Warwick Diabetes Care, which was launched in November 2000 to provide diabetes education for health care professionals throughout the UK. To date, over 4000 health care professionals in the UK have obtained the Warwick Certificate in Diabetes Care.

Dr Gadsby has been active in the RCGP and has been a member of Midland Faculty Board since 1982. He was Vice Chairman from 1994–96, Chairman from 1996–99, and was a member of the RCGP Council from 1994–99.

Acknowledgements

I would like to thank Dr Rodger Charlton for all his help and editorial advice in writing this book.

INTRODUCTION

The Diabetes National Service Framework (NSF) was different from previously published NSFs. It was the first to be in two parts, an initial Standards document published in 2001 and a second Delivery Strategy document which was published in January 2003. The diabetes NSF lacks the large number of detailed milestones and implementation points that previous NSFs had contained.

The quality payment framework included in the new GP contract, which was accepted by the profession in the summer of 2003, gives both detailed process and quality targets that were missing in the diabetes NSF. These quality targets will inevitably become the main drivers for diabetes care delivery in general practice.

There are a good number of diabetes textbooks available today. However, few are specifically targeted at the GP, practice nurse and community diabetes team. There are even fewer that take the delivery of quality diabetes care, as outlined in the quality framework of the new GP contract, as the main focus of attention. The chapters of this book cover in detail each of the 18 quality indicators. The background and evidence base from trials and guidelines is given, along with pragmatic guidance on how to deliver care in order to fulfil the targets. References are included so that original sources can be checked out by those who want to follow the arguments in detail.

There is a paradox inherent in assessing the delivery of quality diabetes care through fulfilling indicators of process and quality. The NSF documents very strongly commend the ideas of patient education, choice and empowerment. There are people living with diabetes who are educated and empowered and who choose, for example, not to run their glycaemic control at a level of an HbA1c of 7.4%, but rather at something a little higher. HbA1c levels in the range 7.5–7.8% suit them and their lifestyle better. There is also the paradox that getting a person to reduce their HbA1c from 7.5% to 7.3% hits a target, and 'targets means points' and 'points means money'; but that sort of drop is likely to be of little clinical significance! However, getting a person to drop their HbA1c from 10.5% to 9% earns no points and no money but is very significant in reducing the risk of adverse outcomes.

Despite these concerns, these quality indicators and the quality payments based on them, are here to stay. This book enables everyone working in community diabetes care to put the quality framework in context and gives readers the information and advice to enable them to deliver quality diabetes care.

1 QUALITY INDICATORS IN THE NEW GP CONTRACT

Background

In the supporting documentation for the new GP contract[1] the authors note that, under the old contract, volume rather than quality was the main emphasis. It is stressed that the new contract addresses this imbalance through introducing a Quality and Outcomes Framework based on best evidence. High achievement against these quality standards is encouraged and this will be reflected in the considerable financial rewards granted to practices that perform well.

Payments to prepare for entering the Quality and Outcomes Framework were guaranteed to all practices in 2003/4. Thereafter resources will rise rapidly. The Department of Health states that the Quality and Outcomes Framework represents a first for any large health system in any country, in that GP practices will be systematically rewarded on the basis of the quality of care delivered to patients.

Calculating payments

The precise details of each practice's payments under the diabetes quality and outcomes framework is still being finalised. Recognition of high practice diabetes prevalence is being recognised.

The sum received by the practice will be:

The square root of (prevalence of diabetes in the practice/nationally agreed diabetes prevalence)
multiplied by
(practice list size/average practice list size)
multiplied by
(number of points obtained for diabetes)
multiplied by
(that year's value for points).

The quality framework

The framework contains four domains. Each domain contains a range of areas described by key indicators. The indicators describe different aspects of performance. The four domains are:

- clinical
- organisational
- additional services
- patient experience.

There are a maximum of 1050 points across all four domains that can be attained.

The clinical domain contains ten disease areas, for which there are a maximum of 550 points.

The diabetes area, has a maximum of 99 points (approximately 10% of the total points available) spread across 18 clinical indicators (see Table 1.1). The only other clinical area with more points (121) is that of coronary heart disease (CHD) including left ventricular dysfunction (LVD). This signifies the importance of diabetes.

Table 1.1 Diabetes clinical indicators

Indicator	Points	Maximum threshold
Records		
DM 1. The practice can produce a register of all patients with diabetes mellitus	6	
Ongoing Management		
DM 2. The percentage of patients with diabetes whose notes record BMI in the previous 15 months	3	90%
DM 3. The percentage of patients with diabetes in whom there is a record of smoking status in the previous 15 months, except those who have never smoked where smoking status should be recorded once	3	90%

Indicator	Points	Maximum threshold
DM 4. The percentage of patients with diabetes who smoke and whose notes contain a record that smoking cessation advice or referral to a specialist service, where available, has been offered in the last 15 months	5	90%
DM 5. The percentage of diabetic patients who have a record of HbA1c or equivalent in the previous 15 months	3	90%
DM 6. The percentage of patients with diabetes in whom the last HbA1c is 7.4 or less (or equivalent test/reference range depending on local laboratory) in last 15 months	16	50%
DM 7. The percentage of patients with diabetes in whom the last HbA1c is 10 or less (or equivalent test/reference range depending on local laboratory) in last 15 months	11	85%
DM 8. The percentage of patients with diabetes who have a record of retinal screening in the previous 15 months	5	90%
DM 9. The percentage of patients with diabetes with a record of the presence or absence of peripheral pulses in the previous 15 months	3	90%
DM 10. The percentage of patients with diabetes with a record of neuropathy testing in the previous 15 months	3	90%
DM 11. The percentage of patients with diabetes who have a record of blood pressure in the past 15 months	3	90%
DM 12. The percentage of patients with diabetes in whom the last blood pressure is 145/85 or less	17	55%

Indicator	Points	Maximum threshold
DM 13. The percentage of patients with diabetes who have a record of microalbuminuria testing in the previous 15 months (exception reporting for patients with proteinuria)	3	90%
DM 14. The percentage of patients with diabetes who have a record of serum creatinine testing in the previous 15 months	3	90%
DM 15. The percentage of patients with diabetes with proteinuria or microalbuminuria who are treated with ACE inhibitors (or A2 antagonists)	3	70%
DM 16. The percentage of patients with diabetes who have a record of total cholesterol in the previous 15 months	3	90%
DM 17. The percentage of patients with diabetes whose last measured total cholesterol within the previous 15 months is 5 or less	6	60%
DM 18. The percentage of patients with diabetes who have had influenza immunisation in the preceding 1 September to 31 March	3	85%

People with diabetes may also have co-morbidities and complications that mean they fit into other clinical areas too, such as the hypertension, CHD and stroke. This will mean that work done in smoking cessation, blood pressure recording and control, and cholesterol recording and control will also count towards points in these other clinical areas.

The diabetes quality targets cover structure, process and outcome as shown opposite.

Box 1.1   Distribution of the 99 points for diabetes

Structure (6 points)	– practice diabetes register
Process (35 points)	– completing various tasks of clinical management
Outcome (58 points)	– demonstrating that people with diabetes achieve good standards of care

Basis for providing quality diabetes care – structured care and regular review

There is clear evidence that regular structured review in the management of people with diabetes is vital to achieving targets and optimising care. More people achieve glycosylated haemoglobin (HbA1c) and blood pressure targets in primary care systems where there is a system of regular recall and review.[2]

Structured care and regular review in primary care are central elements in both parts of the Diabetes NSF,[3-4] and are supported by NICE recommendations and Diabetes UK.[5] Further to this, they now form the basis for the new GP contract's diabetes quality payments system.

Practice infrastructure to deliver quality payments

Staff and dedicated diabetes time

Many practices in the UK run diabetes clinics in which practice nurses, with special training and expertise in diabetes care, recall and review people with diabetes. Such clinics are supervised by the GP partner in the practice who has an interest in diabetes care. In practices with small numbers of people with diabetes, dedicated diabetes clinics may be impractical and specific diabetes time may be best provided in specially designated slots in ordinary surgery times. It is vital that staff providing diabetes care are appropriately skilled. There are a number of excellent diabetes education and training programmes available in the UK that enable a health care professional to gain certification of training through certificates, diplomas and master's degrees in diabetes.

Diabetes register

One of the basic building blocks for running such a clinic is a diabetes register. In the vast majority of practices in the UK this is an electronic register. This is covered in detail in chapter three.

Clinic template

Many practice clinical computer systems contain a diabetes clinic template that automatically uses the appropriate Read codes for recording care. These need to be modified to ensure that they record care information by designated Read codes in a form that will correlate with the quality indicators in the new contract. A diabetes dataset has been developed and is being modified to allow accurate recording of the various items of clinical care that need to be recorded in order to document care which qualifies for the contract quality payments. In most GP diabetes programmes blood tests are requested two weeks before clinic attendance, so that this information is available on the clinic day. Many systems receive test results from the local laboratory by electronic download. These test results are then posted into the diabetes clinical template.

Frequency of review

This clearly depends on the needs of the particular individual. When someone is newly diagnosed their clinical condition may mean that they need reviewing very frequently until their glycaemic control is optimised. Once a person is stabilised and targets for glycaemia and blood pressure have been optimised, routine review every six months is usual.

Payment for the diabetes quality indicators

There are 18 indicators (Table 1.1) in the diabetes quality payment structure. Points are earned for each of them up to a total maximum number of 99 points. Points have a monetary value which will go up annually following the implementation of the new GP contract on the first of April 2004. In the first year the value is expected to be £75 per point = maximum earnings of £7425 in the first year.

A proportion of this is paid according to the practice list size. Set-up monies have been made available to support practices as they work in order to ensure that they have the clinical systems in place for delivering the quality payments. The initial part of the payment is an aspirational payment, approximately one-third of the full potential payment. Practices will be asked what level of quality points they are aiming to gain. Final payments will be made, verified for April 2005, when the actual number of points attained is calculated.

For indicators two to 18 there is a minimum threshold of 25%, and a defined maximum threshold with a number of points allocated for achieving that maximum.

The following example illustrates how payments are calculated for the percentage threshold achieved.

Box 1.2 Indicator 11 example

Indicator 11   Measure of recorded blood pressure

Minimum threshold = 25%

Maximum threshold to achieve full three points = 90%

The practice has to have a recording of blood pressure in the past 15 months for at least 25% of its registered people with diabetes before points can be scored. If 90% or more of such patients have had a blood pressure recording in the previous 15 months it will score three points.

For a percentage between 25 and 90 a proportion of the three points will be earned. The points earned for any percentage above the minimum can be worked out using the formula:

$$\frac{\text{Actual \% } - \text{Minimum \%}}{\text{Maximum \% } - \text{Minimum \%}} \times \text{points available}$$

Say 70% of the registered patients had a blood pressure recording in the past 15 months. Points scored would be:

$$\frac{70-25}{90-25} \times 3 \quad = \quad \frac{45}{65} \times 3 \quad = 2.08 \text{ points}$$

The calculations needed to translate percentages obtained into points gained will be done electronically as part of a software program.

Read codes to be used for recording diabetes information for quality indicators

Read codes are made up of mixtures of letters and numbers. They have been designed to provide a code for all the diagnoses, conditions, symptoms, treatments, and procedures that are encountered in primary care. They have been refined and expanded over time, and are now in a five digit version. New codes are being added to fulfil the requirements of the quality framework, including new exclusion codes. The precise codes in some areas are still being delineated so the summary list opposite can only be provisional.

GP clinical computer system software is being updated by the major providers, to contain the new Read codes that will give automatic encoding when fields in the practice diabetes clinic template are completed. The list opposite will need to be used and referred to as the clinical chapters of this book are read through.

Table 1.2 Read codes

The practice should search for all patients on repeat prescriptions for insulin, oral hypoglycaemics, and blood and urine monitoring sticks

Insulin dependent DM	C108
Non-insulin dependent DM	C109
Impaired glucose tolerance	R102-2

The new codes are:

Type 1 DM	C10E
Type 2 DM	C10F

GMS Contract Codes

The indicators refer to patients with both Type 1 and Type 2 diabetes.

Diabetes (DM) Indicator 1

The practice can produce a register of all patients with diabetes mellitus

Diabetes mellitus	C10%
Type 1 diabetes mellitus	C10E
Type 2 diabetes mellitus	C10F

Diabetes (DM) Indicator 2

The percentage of patients with diabetes whose notes record BMI in the previous 15 months

BMI recorded	22K If value is added via template, Read code not required

Diabetes (DM) Indicator 3

The percentage of patients with diabetes in whom there is a record of smoking status in the previous 15 months, except those who have never smoked where smoking status should be recorded once

Never smoked tobacco	1371
Ex-smoker	137S
Current smoker	137R

Diabetes (DM) Indicator 4

The percentage of patients with diabetes who smoke and whose notes contain a record that smoking cessation advice or referral to a specialist service, where available, has been offered in the last 15 months

Smoking cessation advice	8CAL
Health ed smoking	6791

Diabetes (DM) Indicator 5

The percentage of patients with diabetes who have a record of HbA_{1c} or equivalent in the previous 15 months

HbA_{1c} – diabetic control	42W%
HbA_{1c} level	44TB

Diabetes (DM) Indicator 6

The percentage of patients with diabetes in whom the last HbA_{1c} is 7.4 or less (or equivalent test/reference range depending on local laboratory) in last 15 months

HbA_{1c} level	numeric value

Diabetes (DM) Indicator 7

The percentage of patients with diabetes in whom the last HbA_{1c} is 10 or less (or equivalent test/reference range depending on local laboratory) in last 15 months

HbA_{1c} level	numeric value

Diabetes (DM) Indicator 8

The percentage of patients with diabetes who have a record of retinal screening in the previous 15 months

Diabetic retinal screening	68A7
Fundoscopy normal	31280
Fundoscopy abnormal	31281
Fundoscopy – diabetic check	66AD

Diabetes (DM) Indicator 9

The percentage of patients with diabetes with a record of the presence or absence of peripheral pulses in the previous 15 months

Pulses right	24E%
O/E – right foot pulses present	24EB
O/E – Absent right foot pulses	24EA
Pulses left	24F%
O/E – left foot pulses present	24FB
O/E – Absent left foot pulses	24FA

Diabetes (DM) Indicator 10

10g monofil sens R foot normal	29BB
10g monofil sens R foot abnormal	29B9

The percentage of patients with diabetes with a record of neuropathy testing in the previous 15 months

10g monofil sens L foot normal	29BC
10g monofil sens L foot abnormal	29BA
Vibration sense R foot abnormal	29H4
Vibration sense R foot normal	29H5
Vibration sense L foot abnormal	29H6
Vibration sense L foot normal	29H7

Diabetes (DM) Indicator 11

The percentage of patients with diabetes who have a record of the blood pressure in the past 15 months

O/E – blood pressure reading	246

Diabetes (DM) Indicator 12

The percentage of patients with diabetes in whom the last blood pressure is 145/85 or less

Blood pressure	numeric value

Diabetes (DM) Indicator 13

The percentage of patients with diabetes who have a record of microalbuminuria testing in the previous 15 months (exception reporting for patients with proteinuria)

Urine microalbumin	46W
Urine microalbumin positive	46W0

Urine microalbumin negative	46W1
Urine albumin:creatinine ratio	46TC
24-h urine protein excretion test	46N5

Diabetes (DM) Indicator 14

The percentage of patients with diabetes who have a record of serum creatinine testing in the previous 15 months

Serum creatinine	44J3%

Diabetes (DM) Indicator 15

The percentage of patients with diabetes with proteinuria or microalbuminuria who are treated with ACE inhibitors (or A2 antagonists)

Albuminuria (diagnosis)	R1100
Microalbuminuria (diagnosis)	R1103

Prescribed drugs will be picked up on drug search

ACE inhibitors contraindicated	8I28
ACE inhibitor not indicated	8I64
ACE inhibitor declined	8I3D
ACE inhibitors caus adv eff therap use	U60C4
A2 antagonist contraindicated	8I2H
A2 antagonist declined	8I3
A2 antagonist adverse effect therap use	U60CB
H/O: ACE inhibitor allergy	14LM
ACE inhibitor not tolerated	8I74
H/O: A2 antagonist allergy	14LN
A2 antagonist not indicated	8I6C
A2 antagonist not tolerated	8I75

Diabetes (DM) Indicator 16

The percentage of patients with diabetes who have a record of total cholesterol in the previous 15 months

Serum cholesterol	44P

Diabetes (DM) Indicator 17

The percentage of patients with diabetes whose last measured total cholesterol within the previous 15 months is 5 mmol/l or less

Total cholesterol measurement	44PH

Diabetes (DM) Indicator 18

The percentage patients with diabetes who have a record of influenza immunisation in the preceding 1 September to 31 March

Influenza vaccination	65E
Influenza vac contraindicated	8I2F
No consent – influenza immun	68NE
Influenza vaccination declined	9OX5
H/O: Influenza vaccine allergy	14LJ
Influenza vaccine not indicated	8I6D

Exception reporting

Exception reporting allows the practice to exclude individual patients from the disease indicators in particular circumstances. These are:

Patients exempted from the whole clinical area

- patients who have been recorded as refusing to attend a review, who have been invited on at least three occasions during the preceding 12 months
- patients for whom it is not appropriate to review the chronic disease parameters due to specific circumstances, e.g. extreme frailty or terminal illness or severe dementia
- where a patient does not agree to investigation and treatment (and, after a reasonable discussion or written advice, they have given their informed dissent) and this dissent has been recorded in the medical notes.

Patients exempted from one clinical indicator only (if a valid Read code is used)

- patients on maximum tolerated doses of medication whose level of outcome remains suboptimal
- patients for whom prescribing a medication is not clinically appropriate, e.g. those who have an allergy, another contraindication or who have experienced an adverse reaction
- where a patient has not tolerated a medication
- where a patient does not agree to investigation and treatment (and, after a reasonable discussion or written advice, they have given their informed dissent) and this dissent has been recorded in the medical notes
- where the patient has a supervening condition which makes treatment of their condition inappropriate, e.g. cholesterol reduction where the patient has liver disease

- where an investigative service or secondary care service is unavailable.

Patients exempted automatically from any of the indicators by reporting software

- patients newly diagnosed within the practice with diabetes or who have recently registered with the practice, who should have measurements made within three months and delivery of clinical standards within nine months, e.g. blood pressure or cholesterol measurements within target levels.

Box 1.3   Diabetes exception codes

9h41	Excepted from diabetes quality indictors: Patient unsuitable
9h42	Excepted from diabetes quality indicators: Informed dissent
8BL2	Patient on maximal tolerated therapy for diabetes

References

1. NHS Confederation, British Medical Association. *New GMS Contract 2003: Investing in General Practice.* London: BMA, March 2003 www.bma.org
2. Olivarius N de Fine, Beck-Nielsen H, Andreasen AH *et al.* Randomised controlled trial of structured personal care of type 2 diabetes mellitus. *BMJ* 2001; **323:** 970–5
3. Department of Health. *National Service Framework for Diabetes: Standards.* London: HMSO, 2001 www.dh.gov.uk/assetRoot/04/05/89/38/04058938.pdf (accessed 28 Sept 2004)
4. Department of Health. *National Service Framework for Diabetes: Delivery Strategy.* London: HMSO, December 2002 www.dh.gov.uk/assetRoot/04/03/28/23/04032823.pdf (accessed 28 Sept 2004)
5. Diabetes UK. *Recommendations for the management of diabetes in primary care.* 2nd ed. London: Diabetes UK, October 2000

2 DELIVERING QUALITY DIABETES CARE – UNDERLYING ISSUES

Empowerment

The Diabetes National Service Framework (NSF): Standards,[1] emphasises the need to develop a patient-centred diabetes service in which health professionals working together in teams, educate and empower people with diabetes to care for their condition. Standard 3 specifically deals with empowerment. It states:

> All children, young people and adults with diabetes will receive a service which encourages partnership in decision making, supports them in managing their diabetes and helps them adopt and maintain a healthy lifestyle. This will be reflected in an agreed and shared plan in an appropriate format and language. Where appropriate, parents and carers should be fully engaged in this process.

Professional relationships in the care of diabetic patients have altered over the past twenty years. The traditional model of a powerful paternalistic doctor who dictates treatment, and a subservient patient who listens and obeys, has changed. Now the model is of sharing information between equals: a health care professional and a person living with diabetes, mutually negotiate a management plan and share treatment and care goals, and self-management helps to achieve these goals. The Diabetes NSF in both its sections clearly upholds this view of patient empowerment.

The new GP contract's diabetes quality framework outlines a series of evidenced-based process and quality indicators that the practice needs to achieve in order to gain quality points, and points translate into income for the practice. Is this process compatible with patient empowerment?

The answer is that it ought to be! When the benefits

of good glycaemic control, good blood pressure control and good control of cholesterol have been clearly explained, the person with diabetes can work at the aspects of diet, exercise and concordance with treatment that will enable the targets to be met. When the person with diabetes does not understand the benefits of a course of action they are less likely to comply. However, empowerment could lead to some people choosing not to push themselves to reach a specific target, as the following case history illustrates.

Case history

Mr FT is 36 and has had Type 1 diabetes for 21 years and has four insulin injections daily. He works as a travelling salesman in the food industry. He has an excellent knowledge of his diabetes and uses his skills to vary his insulin doses with his varying levels of exercise and food intake.

He is very frightened of hypoglycaemic attacks and feels that he is beginning to lose his awareness of impending hypoglycaemia. He knows evidence shows that tight control of his blood glucose levels will reduce his risk of microvascular and macrovascular complications, but at the expense of an increased risk of hypoglycaemia. He therefore chooses to maintain an HbA1c level of 7.8%, which he feels for him is the best compromise between reducing risk of complications and having a negligible risk of hypoglycaemia.

This person chooses not to aim to achieve the new contract HbA1c target of 7.4%, for very good personal reasons. This should be documented and an exclusion code used so that the case is not counted as part of the population from which the 50% at or below an HbA1c of 7.4 is calculated.

What is the evidence that empowerment is of benefit?

Patient satisfaction and knowledge improve when lifestyle interventions in Type 2 diabetes are delivered by primary care staff who have been trained to take a patient-centred approach.[2] However, improvements in patient knowledge do not always result in the achievement of better diabetes control, as measured by improvement in HbA1c levels.

There is evidence from studies in children and young adults with Type 1 diabetes that interventions that promote education and diabetes-specific coping skills have a positive effect on diabetes knowledge, improved management and glycaemic control.[3]

Actions for primary care
1. Encourage empowerment by clearly explaining the advantages and any possible disadvantages of reaching diabetes quality targets.
2. If individuals, for personal reasons, do not to want to aim to achieve specific diabetes quality targets, they can be excluded using the appropriate Read code. The reason for using the exclusion code needs to be clearly documented in the clinical record.

Concordance with therapy

The problem of patients not complying with treatment was first recorded over 2000 years ago when Hippocrates advised the physician 'to be alert to the faults of the patients which make them lie about their taking of the medicines prescribed and when things go wrong, refuse to confess that they have not been taking their medicine.'[4] In a retrospective cohort study from Scotland,[5] 2920 subjects with at least 12 months' prescriptions for oral hypoglycaemic agents were identified, and their adherence to treatment was estimated using data gathered from dispensed prescriptions. Adequate adherence to treatment, defined as dispensed doses of at least 90% of doses prescribed, was found in only 31% on sulphonylurea monotherapy and 34% on metformin monotherapy. There were significant linear trends of poorer adherence with each increase in daily number of tablets taken, and increase in co-medication.

There are several reasons why people may not take their tablets as prescribed including:

- lack of education or understanding regarding appropriate self-administration and the importance of daily treatment
- confusion over which tablets to take when. This may especially occur in older people with developing memory loss
- changes in drug or dose regimen
- unpleasant side effects
- physical problems opening the packaging or problems reading the label
- demands of a busy lifestyle.

Actions for primary care

1. Carefully explain to people what each tablet is for, when it should be taken, and the importance of remembering to take each treatment as prescribed.
2. Try to minimise the number of tablets to be taken, and the frequency with which they need to be taken – from a concordance perspective, once-daily treatments are the ideal.
3. Use treatments that have few, if any, side effects wherever possible.
4. Ensure treatments are appropriately packaged and labelling is clear.
5. If a patient regularly forgets whether he or she has taken his/her tablets, consider pre-filled tablet dispensing systems.

Monitoring

People using insulin, whether they have Type 1 or Type 2 diabetes, need to be able to monitor their blood glucose levels. Blood glucose monitoring enables them to vary doses of insulin according to the level of physical activity and eating pattern on a dose by dose basis. This gives much more flexibility in daily living and gives the opportunity for improved overall control.

In Type 2 diabetes treated with oral agents and/or diet alone there is much less consensus about the benefits of blood glucose monitoring. A meta-analysis of studies on self-monitoring in Type 2 diabetes failed to demonstrate the effectiveness of blood glucose monitoring in improving glycaemic control, and failed to demonstrate a difference in diabetes control between blood and urine glucose monitoring.[6]

Blood glucose monitoring technology is progressing quickly and a number of new monitors that require much smaller quantities of blood are being developed. This enables blood samples to be taken from the forearm, and is resulting in the concept of almost painless monitoring'.

In some areas of the UK spending on blood glucose monitoring now exceeds that of insulin itself, and attempts are being made to rationalise prescribing of blood glucose sticks. However, it seems reasonable to support the argument that people with diabetes who are using insulin should be prescribed enough sticks to test as often as they need to. A recent consensus report has suggested guidelines for the rational use of blood glucose monitoring in Type 1 and Type 2 diabetes.[7]

For people with Type 2 diabetes treated with oral agents and/or diet there is an argument that if they regularly blood glucose monitor until their HbA1c stabilises they will more quickly learn the relationship between exercise, food intake and blood glucose levels, than those people who choose not to monitor their blood glucose levels. Once the HbA1c is stable there is little point, in my opinion, in routinely testing blood glucose levels on a daily basis. However, it is very important to test frequently during times of intercurrent illness to check for low or high blood glucose levels.

Actions for primary care
1. Ensure people using insulin monitor their blood glucose levels as appropriate.
2. Discuss with people newly diagnosed with Type 2 diabetes the advantages of blood glucose monitoring and prescribe equipment if they want to do it.
3. Ensure that everybody who is blood glucose monitoring knows why they are doing it, and are empowered to act on the results.
4. Discourage people from unthinking, routine blood glucose monitoring.

Ethnic issues

Epidemiology

There is a fourfold increased risk of Type 2 diabetes amongst people from South Asia (India, Sri Lanka, Pakistan and Bangladesh) living in the UK as compared with Europeans.[8] Type 2 diabetes also seems to develop in South Asians about ten years earlier than in Europeans and renal and cardiac complications are encountered more commonly. Although genetic factors are important, the increased risk of Type 2 diabetes is strongly associated with increasing central obesity and insulin resistance.

The World Health Organization has recommended lower levels of BMI as desirable in South Asians, and has classified overweight as a BMI greater than 23 in this group (compared with 25 in Europeans).

Preventing diabetes and obesity

The particular educational needs of the South Asian community need to be addressed, with programmes on healthy lifestyle, improved diet, and increased physical activity, designed to reduce obesity, and hence reducing the risks of developing Type 2 diabetes. These programmes need to be culturally sensitive and be available in appropriate languages. The use of Asian link workers to promote such programmes is being tested in some areas of the UK. Similar educational programmes are needed for people who develop Type 2 diabetes.

Treating people from ethnic minority backgrounds

It is vital that the educational programmes needed for people with newly diagnosed and established diabetes be culturally sensitive and available in appropriate languages. Translators may be needed to assist in consultations with people who cannot speak English. Fasting during the hours of daylight during Ramadan for Muslims may need special advice and management.

Actions for primary care
1. Practices which have large numbers of registered patients from a South Asian background may have three or four times as many people on their diabetes register, causing huge workload implications.
2. Obesity needs to be defined at lower levels of BMI in these populations.
3. Culturally sensitive education will be needed in appropriate languages.

Special groups – older people

Background

The definition of older people is arbitrary but one that can be used is to define people as 'old' when they are over 75 years of age and 'very old' if they are over 85 years of age. Type 2 diabetes is a condition that most commonly occurs in middle aged and older people. In many practices, over 50% of people on the practice diabetes register will be 65 years old and over.

One of the main concerns in implementing the quality framework for diabetes in older people is likely to be 'how hard should health care professionals strive to get old and very old people to achieve the quality targets for glycaemic control, blood pressure and cholesterol'. The concern might be that zealous striving after blood pressure and HbA1c targets might result in impairment of quality of life by increasing the risks of hypotension and hypoglycaemia.

The evidence base

In the UKPDS glycaemic control study newly diagnosed people with Type 2 diabetes were enrolled up to the age of 65. They were followed for a mean of ten years. So it can be suggested that there is an evidence base for tight glycaemic control up to the age of 75 years.[9] Studies carried out specifically in older people tend to be descriptive rather than true randomised controlled trials. The heart protection study (HPS) recruited people up to 80 years and followed them for a mean of four years. It can therefore be suggested that there is an evidence base for cholesterol lowering with a statin up to 80–84 years.[10] Several trials of blood pressure lowering treatment in general populations have recruited people up to age 78 or 80 years, so it can also be argued that there is an evidence base for blood pressure lowering up to the age of around 80 years of age.

However, those enrolled into clinical trials tend to be relatively fit, healthy people who have a single specific disease – the one being studied in the trial. This doesn't fit the picture of many of the old or very old people with Type 2 diabetes seen in primary care.

Fit, independent and frail older people

It is possible to divide old and very old people into two broad categories:

1. Those who have Type 2 diabetes as their only significant disease and are otherwise healthy and living independently.

   Where evidence is lacking, treat to targets set for younger people, in consultation with the individual. Around one third of individuals fall into this group, based on data from a large community study in Wales conducted during the 1990s where objective measures of dependency were based on Barthel activities of daily living (ADL) score, Extended ADL score and minimental state examination score.[11]

2. Those who have significant co-morbidities, e.g. arthritis, high dependency levels, or significant dementia.

Around two thirds fall into this group.[11] Practical care for people in this group would be to ensure symptomatic control, avoid hypoglycaemia and intensive monitoring, in consultation with the individual and their carers. In relation to the Quality and Outcomes Framework contained in the GP contract, the exclusion codes can then be used for those in whom it is deemed that achieving the targets would not be medically advisable.

Actions for primary care

1. After discussion and with the agreement of the person, treat to target those old and very old people who only have Type 2 diabetes and who are independent and fit.

2. After discussion and with the agreement of the person (where possible) and their carers, frail elderly people with significant co-morbidities should be treated to keep them free of glycaemic symptoms, and to give them as good a quality of life as possible. Use the exclusion codes to ensure that the practice is not penalised for not reaching the targets in this group of frail elderly people.

Children and adolescents

Background

Most children and young people with diabetes registered with a practice will have Type 1 diabetes. The repeat prescribing of insulin will continue to take place in primary care, but young patients are likely to receive their detailed management and care from a hospital paediatric service. Information on diabetes control from hospital letters will need to be entered on the practice diabetes database. Support for the parents and carers of children with Type 1 diabetes is vital, and local peer support groups can be very helpful in providing this.

Diabetes control can deteriorate during puberty and adolescence for a variety of reasons. Teenage rebellion can result in insulin injections being overlooked with resulting hyperglycaemia with risk of ketoacidosis. The transition from paediatric care to adult diabetic clinic care needs to be handled sensitively and a number of hospital centres run special transition clinics staffed by members of both paediatric and adult diabetes services to try to ensure this goes as smoothly as possible.

A new NICE guideline on the management of children and young people with Type 1 diabetes was launched in 2004.[12] Retinopathy screening, blood pressure measurement, and microalbuminuria screening are being recommended from age 12 onwards. Exclusion codes for these processes will need to be used for those younger than 12 years.

There is evidence of increasing numbers of children and adolescents being diagnosed with Type 2 diabetes, initially in the USA, but more recently in the UK.[13] Obesity is a common finding in these young people, as is decreased physical activity. Many of those diagnosed in the UK come from the South Asian community and have a positive family history of Type 2 diabetes. Their treatment and management follows similar lines to adults with Type 2 diabetes, but referral to specialist services will be helpful to try to help with the significant psycho–social impact of the diabetes and obesity.

Actions for primary care
1. Ensure that children and young people with Type 1 diabetes are receiving optimal care from hospital clinics.
2. Refer teenagers with Type 2 diabetes for the specialised care they will need to manage their diabetes and obesity.
3. Use exclusion codes for retinopathy, blood pressure and microalbuminuria indicators for the under 12s.

Hierarchy of evidence and grading of recommendations

The following definitions are used in this book for the evidence-based grading of recommendations. They are based on the ones used in the development of NICE guidelines.[12]

Table 2.1 Definitions for evidence-based grading of recommendations

Classification of evidence	
Evidence level	Description
Ia:	evidence from meta-analysis of randomised controlled trials
Ib:	evidence from at least one randomised controlled trial
IIa:	evidence from at least one controlled study without randomisation
IIb:	evidence from at least one other type of quasi-experimental study
III:	evidence from non-experimental descriptive studies, such as comparative studies, correlation studies and case-control studies
IV:	evidence from expert committee reports or opinions and/or clinical experience of respected authorities
Grading of recommendations	
A	directly based on category I evidence
B	directly based on category II evidence, or extrapolated recommendation from category I evidence
C	directly based on category III evidence, or extrapolated recommendation from category I or II evidence
D	directly based on category IV evidence, or extrapolated recommendation from category I, II or III evidence

References
1. Department of Health. *National Service Framework for Diabetes: Standards.* London: HMSO, 2001 www.dh.gov.uk/assetRoot/04/05/89/38/04058938.pdf (accessed 28 Sept 2004)
2. Kinmonth AL, Woodcock A, Griffin S, Spiegal N, Campbell MJ. Randomised

controlled trial of patient-centred care of diabetes in general practice: impact on current wellbeing and future disease risk. *BMJ* 1998; **317**: 1202–8

3. Hampton SE, Skinner TC, Hart J *et al.* Effects of educational and psychological interventions for adolescents with diabetes: a systematic review. *Health Technol Assess* 2001; **5**: 1–79

4. Sawyer S. Adherence: Whose Responsibility? In: *A Decade of Coordinated Asthma Management in Australia.* Melbourne: National Asthma Campaign, 1998, pp. 9–10

5. Donnan PT, MacDonald TM, Morris AD for the DARTS/MEMO Collaboration. *Diabet Med* 2002; **19**: 279–84

6. Coster S, Guilliford MC, Seed PT, Powrie JK, Swaminathan R. Self-monitoring in Type 2 diabetes: a meta-analysis. *Diabet Med* 2000; **17**: 755–61

7. Owens D, Barnett AH, Pickup J *et al.* Blood glucose self-monitoring in type 1 and type 2 diabetes: reaching a multidisciplinary consensus. *Diabetes and Primary Care* 2004; **6**: 8–16

8. Chowdhury TA, Grace C, Kopelman P. Preventing diabetes in south Asians. *BMJ* 2003; **327**: 1059–60

9. United Kingdom Prospective Diabetes Study UKPDS 33. Intensive blood glucose control with sulphonylureas or insulin compared with conventional treatment and risk of complications in patients with Type 2 diabetes. *Lancet* 1998; **352**: 837–53

10. Heart Protection Study Group. MRC/BHF Heart Protection Study of cholesterol lowering with simvastatin in 20,536 high-risk individuals: a randomised placebo-controlled trial. *Lancet* 2002; **360**: 7–22

11. Sinclair AJ, Bayer AJ. All Wales Research in Elderly (AWARE) Diabetes Study, 121/3040. London: Department of Health, 1998

12. NICE. Type 1 diabetes: diagnosis and management of Type 1 diabetes in children and young people. London: NICE, 15 July 2004 www.nice.org.uk/page.aspx?o=213575 (accessed 19 Oct 2004)

13. Gadsby R. Epidemiology of diabetes. *Advanced Drug Reviews* 2002; **54**: 1165–72

3 REGISTERS, DIABETES DIAGNOSIS AND CLASSIFICATION

> **Diabetes quality indicator 1 (DM1)**
> *The practice can produce a register of all patients with diabetes mellitus* = 6 points

Background

A register of all people who have been diagnosed as having diabetes mellitus and who are registered with the practice is a fundamental requirement for achieving quality payments under the new contract. Practice clinical computer systems have an electronic diabetes register and as soon as a person is newly diagnosed with diabetes they can be added to the register. The C10 Read code signifies diabetes mellitus. It is vital that only people with properly diagnosed diabetes are allocated with C10 and entered onto the register.

Evidence

There is clear evidence that regular structured review in the management of people with diabetes is vital to achieving targets and optimising care. More people achieve HbA1c targets and blood pressure targets in primary care systems where there is a system of regular recall and review.[1]

Structured care and regular review in primary care are central parts of the Diabetes NSF, and are supported by NICE recommendations and Diabetes UK.[2-3] There is evidence that clinical outcomes are best when computerised recall systems based on registers of people with diabetes are used.[4]

The next section details how the diagnosis of diabetes is made so that the patient can be entered onto the practice diabetes register.

Diagnosing diabetes

The new World Health Organization (WHO) criteria for diagnosing diabetes were adopted in the UK on 1 June 2000.[5] These give the criteria for diagnosing diabetes on fasting or random blood glucose measurements.

On fasting blood results (see Fig 3.1)

Diabetes is diagnosed as a fasting plasma glucose of 7 mmol and above.

Fig. 3.1   Diagnosis of diabetes: Fasting plasma glucose

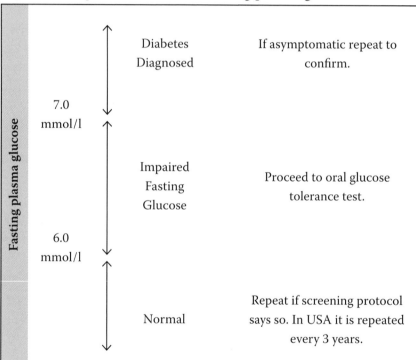

On random or post glucose challenge results (see Fig 3.2)

The blood glucose level for diagnosing diabetes on a random plasma glucose or a post 75g glucose challenge is 11.1 mmol and above.

Fig. 3.2   Diagnosis of diabetes: Oral glucose tolerance test (OGTT – plasma glucose after 2 hours following a 75g glucose load)

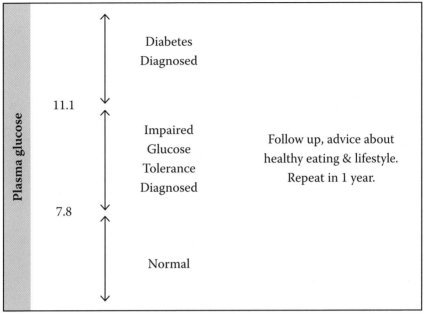

In patients who are asymptomatic

Two abnormal blood glucose measurements diagnostic of diabetes must be obtained.

Impaired fasting glucose

Under these new criteria those with fasting glucose levels below 6 mmol are classified as normal and those with levels between 6 and 7 are classified as having impaired fasting glucose (IFG) (Figure 3.1).

If IFG is diagnosed, Diabetes UK recommends that an OGTT is performed[5] to find out whether they might have blood glucose levels diagnostic of diabetes. To perform an OGTT a person has a fasting blood specimen taken and is then given 75 gm of glucose orally. A further blood glucose estimation is taken two hours later.

If the two-hour glucose level is 11.1 or above diabetes is diagnosed. If the two-hour level is below 7.8 it is classified as normal, if it is between 7.8 and 11.1 a diagnosis of impaired glucose tolerance (IGT) is made.

These points are illustrated in Figure 3.2. IGT and IFG are together referred to as pre-diabetes.

The diagnosis of diabetes has important medico–legal implications – for example, for driving and insurance – and so diagnostic blood glucose estimations must be obtained from a laboratory with appropriate quality control mechanisms, rather than by hand-held glucose oxidase stick testing measurements.

Diabetes symptoms

The classical symptoms of hyperglycaemia are of polyuria and polydypsia. They commonly occur in people newly presenting with Type 1 diabetes and may be associated with weight loss, nausea, vomiting, ketosis and dehydration.

In Type 2 diabetes symptoms may be absent, or may be very non-specific such as tiredness and lethargy. The classical symptoms of polyuria and polydypsia even when present will not be volunteered but sometimes can only be elucidated by direct questioning. Both the general public and health care professionals may think that such non-specific symptoms reflect the normal ageing process and so the diagnosis of Type 2 diabetes may be overlooked for a long time. Campaigns to alert the general public to the symptoms of diabetes have been instituted from time to time in the UK.[6] Health care professionals need to 'think diabetes' whenever someone presents with non-specific symptoms and to arrange blood glucose testing as appropriate.

Numbers to expect on your diabetes register

My practice has an ethnic mix of 95% Caucasian with 5% from a variety of ethnic minorities and has had a stable list size of 14,500 over the past 30 years. I have seen a rise in numbers on our diabetes register from 1.8% of our total list size in 1985, to 3.2% in 2003. In practices with large numbers of people from ethnic minority backgrounds the diabetes register may comprise up to 12% of the people registered with the practice. Risk factors for obesity include ethnic background and increasing levels of obesity and physical inactivity. So in an 'average' practice in the UK with relatively small numbers of people from ethnic minorities, at least 3% of the practice population are likely to have been diagnosed as having diabetes. This may be lower than 3%, in practices with large numbers of young people on their list – for instance in student health centre practices – and much greater than 3% in practices with larger numbers of older people, and in practices with larger numbers of people from South Asian ethnic minority backgrounds.

It may be that Primary Care Trusts (PCTs) will check the numbers on a practice register with the PCT average, and compare them with the anticipated numbers expected in that particular geographical location.

People with Type 1 diabetes will make up about 10–15% of those on the register, whereas 85–90% will have Type 2 diabetes.

Why is the number of people with diabetes increasing?

The prevalence of Type 2 diabetes is rapidly rising throughout the developed world. The recently published *Diabetes Atlas 2000*[7] estimates that there are currently around 151 million people in the 20–79 age group with diabetes in the world, a global prevalence of 4.6%. Worldwide, the number of people with diabetes is expected to double over the 13-year period 1997–2010 to a total of 221 million. Prevalence rates are expected to rise by 111% in Asia, 93% in Africa, 51% in Europe and 35% in North America in the same period.

The major factors leading to this massive explosion in the number of people developing Type 2 diabetes are obesity and increasingly sedentary lifestyles. As previously mentioned, it is also more common in people from certain ethnic groups including those from Indo-Asia.

Type 2 diabetes is now starting to be diagnosed in teenagers, most of whom are significantly obese. They are likely to manifest the serious complications of diabetes when they are 30–40 years old.[8]

Should you screen for diabetes in your practice?

The Diabetes NSF[9] does not recommend population-based screening for asymptomatic individuals in England at present. It states that those who are known to have a high risk of developing Type 2 diabetes, including people who have been found to have impaired glucose regulation (IGT and IFG) and women with a history of gestational diabetes, should receive follow-up and regular testing. This should also be complemented by advice and support to reduce their risk of developing diabetes, and information to help them recognise the symptoms and signs of diabetes. In addition, it indicates that people with multiple risk factors for diabetes, such as family history, ethnic background, obesity, and increasing age also need advice and support to reduce their risk of developing diabetes, and information about the signs and symptoms of diabetes. It states that opportunistic screening will identify some people who do not know they have the condition.

Research studies are presently underway to try to resolve the question of who should be screened. In one particular study, the Diabetes, Heart Disease and Stroke Screening (DHDS) study, three practices in nine teaching PCTs are screening people with BMIs over 30 for diabetes and heart disease. They are due to report in a couple of years and this research will inform the National Screening Committee's report to the Department of Health, which the NSF states will occur in 2005. Currently, advice would be to opportunistically screen for diabetes in those people who are on the CHD and hypertension registers, and to think diabetes whenever someone presents with vague symptoms of tiredness and lethargy, and arrange for them to have a glucose estimation.

The problem of interpretation of random glucose estimations

The diagnostic criteria for diabetes state that diabetes is diagnosed when a laboratory random glucose estimation is above 11.1 mmol.

It can be very difficult to assign meaning to a random blood glucose measurement of say 7 mmol when such a result is received as part of a general blood screen of full blood count, urea and electrolytes, liver function tests, thyroid function tests and glucose, taken as part of the work-up of someone presenting with vague non-specific symptoms of tiredness and lethargy. The result would have a different meaning if we knew the person had not had anything to eat for six hours before the test than it would have if we knew it had been taken two hours after a high sugar meal! In the former case it would be suggestive of diabetes; in the latter case it would be completely normal.

To be sure of not missing diabetes it could be necessary to proceed to a more accurate screening test, using a fasting glucose estimation, on those with random glucose values of say 6.5 or above. The problem is that a significant proportion of people with a random glucose estimation of 6.5 will have normal fasting levels, and not have diabetes. The difficulties with random glucose values can be side stepped by using the fasting glucose sample as the screen for diabetes whenever possible. It can easily be added to the fasting blood tests taken for lipids in those with CHD and hypertension.

HbA1c estimations are not sensitive or specific enough at present to be part of the diagnostic criteria for diabetes. However, a raised level at diagnosis along with the necessary two abnormal glucose estimations can be thought of as useful confirmatory evidence. Equally, a completely normal HbA1c might lead one to question and perhaps repeat abnormal blood glucose values.

Case history

Mr SW a 56-year-old man with a BMI of 31, attended surgery with symptoms of tiredness and lethargy. Blood tests were carried out that came back from the laboratory marked normal. The random glucose level was 9 mmol. The test had been taken late morning, after an early breakfast. A fasting glucose test was therefore performed and was 6.8 mmol. It was repeated and a result of 6.9 was obtained. In view of the two fasting glucose measurements in the impaired fasting glucose range, an oral glucose tolerance test was requested. The fasting level came back as 6.9 and the two-hour level 13.6 mmol, which confirmed a diagnosis of diabetes, on the basis of one abnormal blood glucose estimation plus symptoms.

Two years later he is well controlled on diet and exercise, and has managed to reduce his BMI to 29.

Possible sources of inaccuracy in the practice diabetes register

The following may be encountered in practice:

- patients diagnosed as having diabetes many years ago, simply through having glycosuria, being included on the register. When their notes are inspected it is found that no diagnostic blood tests were ever performed
- patients with gestational diabetes being put on the diabetes register
- patients with diabetes insipidus being put on the register
- patients with IFG or IGT being wrongly labelled as having diabetes and being put on the register
- patients who are asymptomatic with only one abnormal blood glucose level being diagnosed as having diabetes and being put on the register
- a patient who had an isolated raised blood glucose level during admission for a myocardial infarction and was labelled as having diabetes was put on the register – the OGTT ten weeks after admission was completely normal.

Case history

Mrs JN, a 71-year-old lady with a BMI of 28 with no significant previous medical history, was admitted to hospital with a myocardial infarction. On admission she had a blood glucose result of 14.3 mmol and was started on insulin. She made a full recovery and was discharged on insulin, taking a total dose of 12 units per day. She began to develop signs of hypoglycaemia and had low normal random blood glucose estimations throughout the day. Her insulin was stopped. The results of an oral glucose tolerance test eight weeks after admission showed a fasting level of 5.9 and a two-hour level of 7.2, both of which are normal. Her name was removed from the diabetes register.

The raised blood glucose at the time of admission with a myocardial infarction was presumably just due to stress hyperglycaemia.

It is important to adhere to the correct diagnostic criteria for diabetes and to ensure that the register is accurate.

Actions for primary care

1. Ensure that people with diabetes are accurately diagnosed using the WHO criteria and entered onto the practice diabetes register using the C10 Read code.
2. Ensure that people with just impaired fasting glucose or impaired glucose tolerance do not get entered as having diabetes onto the register but are separately coded.
3. Opportunistically screen people on the practice CHD and hypertension registers for diabetes, using fasting glucose measurements wherever possible.

Summary points

- Use an electronic register in the practice clinical computer system to record all people with diabetes using the C10 Read code.
- The 'average practice' could expect at least 3% of the practice population to have diabetes. This will be considerably more in practices with large numbers of people from Indo-Asian ethnic groups.
- Make sure all people listed on the register fulfil the new diagnostic criteria for diabetes.
- Ensure you have two abnormal blood glucose estimations for asymptomatic individuals.
- Proceed to an OGTT on people with two glucose levels in the IFG range.
- Screen for diabetes opportunistically in people at risk using fasting glucose measurements.
- Take care in interpreting random glucose measurements, and go on to fasting glucose measurements if in doubt.

References

1. Olivarius N de Fine, Beck-Nielsen H, Andreasen AH *et al.* Randomised controlled trial of structured personal care of type 2 diabetes mellitus. *BMJ* 2001; **323**: 970–5
2. Diabetes UK. Recommendations for the management of diabetes in primary care. 2nd ed. London: Diabetes UK, October 2000
3. European Diabetes Policy Group. A desktop guide to diabetes mellitus. *Diabet Med* 1999; **16**: 716–30
4. Griffin S, Kinmonth AL. Systems for routine surveillance for people with diabetes mellitus (Cochrane Review). Cochrane Library 2002; **2**: Oxford: Update Software
5. British Diabetic Association (now Diabetes UK). New Diagnostic Criteria for Diabetes. London: British Diabetic Association, April 2000
6. Singh B, Prescott J, Guy R et al. Effect of advertising on awareness of symptoms of diabetes among the general public: the British Diabetic Association Study. BMJ 1994; **308**: 632–6
7. Diabetes Atlas 2000. Brussels: International Diabetes Federation (IDF), July 2000
8. Rosenbloom JR, Joe JR, Young RS, Winter WE. Emerging epidemic of Type 2 diabetes in youth. *Diabetes Care* 1999; **22**: 345–54
9. Department of Health. National Service Framework for Diabetes: Standards. London: HMSO, 2001 www.dh.gov.uk/assetRoot/04/05/89/38/04058938.pdf (accessed 28 Sept 2004)

4. WEIGHT MANAGEMENT

Diabetes quality indicator 2 (DM2)
The percentage of patients with diabetes whose notes record Body Mass Index (BMI) in the previous 15 months:
Minimum threshold = 25%, maximum threshold to earn full available 3 points = 90%

Background

Obesity is closely associated with the development of Type 2 diabetes. One of the major reasons for the current 'epidemic' of Type 2 diabetes worldwide is the increasing prevalence of obesity worldwide.[1] Reducing weight can delay or prevent diabetes in groups at risk of developing Type 2 diabetes[2-3] and in obese people generally.[4] Weight reduction in overweight individuals is the cornerstone of management of people with Type 2 diabetes.[5] Weighing a person with Type 2 diabetes during visits to the GP practice diabetes clinic is therefore a vital part of ongoing management. Clinical computer systems will calculate the BMI once weight is entered onto the computer if a height measurement is already recorded for that person on the system.

Evidence base from clinical trials

Reducing weight in at-risk populations can prevent the development of Type 2 diabetes

A Finnish study among 522 middle-aged, overweight subjects with impaired glucose tolerance (IGT) – individuals at significantly increased risk for Type 2 diabetes – clearly showed that an active programme of increased physical activity and dietary change can prevent the onset of the disease.[2] When compared with routine care, individualised counselling for life-style changes resulted in an increased level of physical activity, and a significant loss of weight; mean loss of 3.5 ± 5.5kg after two years. This active treatment conferred a 58% reduction in the risk for developing diabetes; the cumulative incidence of diabetes after four years being 11%, compared with 23% in the control group receiving routine care.

Further evidence on the effectiveness of nutrition and exercise therapy in preventing diabetes developing in people with IGT, who are at very significant risk of developing diabetes, comes from the Diabetes Prevention Study from the USA.[3] In this study several thousand people with IGT were divided into groups. One group received a diet and exercise programme that was aimed at achieving a weight reduction of around 7%, and moderate physical activity, for example, brisk walking for 150 minutes per week. People in the active arm of the study had regular one-to-one sessions with their case manager in the first 24 weeks, and then monthly sessions for the remaining period of the study. Fifty per cent of people achieved the weight reduction target at 24 weeks and 74% achieved the exercise target. When compared to the control group who received 'general advice' those in the lifestyle and exercise group reduced their risk of developing diabetes by 58%, exactly the same risk reduction as in the Finnish study.

Preventing diabetes in obese people by lifestyle change and anti-obesity medication

Another approach to reducing the incidence of diabetes that has been tested in a randomised controlled trial has been to use the lipase inhibitor orlistat, which acts locally in the gut to reduce absorption of ingested fat, in combination with lifestyle change. In the XENDOS study carried out in 22 centres in Sweden, 3304 obese individuals – 21% of whom had IGT – were given lifestyle advice and either placebo or orlistat 120mg tds, and were followed for four years. Those receiving orlistat lost on average 6.9kg in weight against 4.1kg on placebo. The cumulative incidence of Type 2 diabetes was

9% in the lifestyle plus placebo group and 6.2% in the lifestyle plus orlistat group, a risk reduction of 37%. This study shows that in an obese population, in which 21% had IGT, orlistat together with lifestyle change over four years resulted in a greater weight loss and a significantly reduced incidence of Type 2 diabetes as compared to intensive lifestyle changes alone. The drug orlistat was well tolerated in the study.[4]

Recommendations from guidelines

The Scottish Intercollegiate Guidelines Network (SIGN) guidelines[5] state that healthy eating is of fundamental importance as part of diabetes health care behaviour and has beneficial effects of weight, metabolic control and general well being. In particular weight control in overweight subjects with diabetes is associated with improved glycaemic control.[6] People with Type 2 diabetes often find weight management to be very difficult. Emphasis as to its importance, and encouragement to lose weight, are therefore vital parts of diabetes education and management.

Education for healthy eating for people with Type 2 diabetes

NICE has published a review on education in diabetes.[7] It recommends that structured patient education is made available to all people with diabetes at the time of initial diagnosis and then as required on an ongoing basis, based on a formal, regular assessment of need.

The document concludes that there is insufficient evidence currently available to recommend a specific type of education or provide guidance on the setting for, or frequency of, education sessions for people newly diagnosed with Type 2 diabetes. However, it states that to achieve maximum effectiveness, educational interventions should reflect established principles of adult learning.

The benefits of education

Research has shown that patient satisfaction and knowledge improve when lifestyle interventions in Type 2 diabetes are delivered by primary care staff who have been trained to take a patient-centred approach.[8]

The NSF states that there is good evidence that structured education can improve knowledge, blood glucose control, weight and dietary management, physical activity and psychological wellbeing, particularly when this is tailored to the needs of the individual.[9]

Education in the practice

Education provides the basis for patient empowerment and self-care concepts that are beginning to take a much more pivotal role in diabetes care. This means that education, often given by practice nurses, will need to become more formalised and documented. It also needs be supported by the provision of suitable literature for the person with diabetes.

The level and pace of learning varies between individuals. Supplying too little information or inundating the person with too much are equally disastrous. Good education techniques include:

- focussing on the person's experience and previous knowledge
- linking specific knowledge or skill with general therapeutic objectives
- trying to enhance the person's understanding.

Education is enhanced if verbal education is backed up by written information. For example, a practice can provide people newly diagnosed as having Type 2 diabetes with the Diabetes UK publication *Diabetes for Beginners, Living with Type 2 Diabetes*. This gives them a comprehensive overview of their condition and helps to introduce them to Diabetes UK.

Programme for diabetes education for people with Type 2 diabetes

Many organisations have developed programmes for diabetes patient education. The International Diabetes Federation has published the International Consensus Standards of Practice for Diabetes Education[10] which outline the key elements and frameworks by which the structure, process and outcome of diabetes education can be assessed. The suggested content of diabetes self-management education from the Education Study Group of the European Association for the Study of Diabetes[11] is outlined in Box 4.1.

Box 4.1 Diabetes education: programme content

- diabetes overview
- stress and psychosocial adjustment
- family involvement and social support
- nutrition
- exercise and activity
- medications
- monitoring and use of results
- relationships between nutrition, exercise, medication and blood glucose levels
- prevention, detection and treatment of chronic complications
- foot, skin and dental care
- behaviour change strategies, goal setting, risk factor reduction and problem solving
- benefits, risks and management options for improving glucose control
- preconception care, pregnancy and gestational diabetes
- use of health care systems and community resources

Healthy eating

An emphasis in diabetes on the concept of healthy eating is important and its adoption by all members of the family will help in patient self-management. A simple written guide (Table 4.1) can reinforce healthy eating messages. Weight reduction in those who are overweight is a vital part of Type 2 diabetes management. Regular weighing and encouragement of weight loss (in those who are overweight), at each practice diabetes visit, can help self-management in this difficult area. Some people also benefit from attendance at peer support groups such as 'weight watchers' and similar groups.

Table 4.1 A simple guide to nutrition and Type 2 diabetes

Eat regularly	• Do not miss meals, aim to have 3 meals a day • Eat 5 portions of fruit and vegetables a day
Avoid added sugar and sugary foods	• Do not add sugar to any food or drink • Avoid all drinks sweetened with sugar, jams, marmalade and honey • Instead use low calorie and sugar free drinks (often labelled as diet drinks). You may use sugar free artificial sweeteners • Avoid sugary biscuits, cakes, sugary puddings or desserts, sweets, chocolates
Eat plenty of fibre	• Good sources of fibre are fibre rich breakfast cereals, whole-grain bread, oats, beans, peas, lentils, fruit, vegetables, potatoes, brown rice, wholemeal pasta
Eat less fat	• Use semi-skimmed or skimmed milk • Cut down on butter, margarine, oil, lard, and cheese • Eat lean meat and remove visible fat • Grill food rather than frying it

Avoid special diabetic products	• For example sweets, biscuits, jams, chocolate – they are usually expensive
Try to be the right weight for your height	• Lose weight if you are overweight

Physical activity

Encouraging physical activity in people with diabetes is a vital part of management, and has been shown to help prevent the onset of diabetes in susceptible individuals.[2–3] It is important that advice about exercise should be realistic, simple, individualised, and enjoyable. Gentle walking for 20 minutes a day is a realistic goal in self-management for many people with diabetes. In parts of the UK 'walking for exercise' schemes have been established where people are invited to join in set walks which are organised and led by local volunteers. Enquiry about, and encouragement of, physical activity at each diabetes clinic visit can help weight loss in the overweight population.

Education and empowerment in Type 1 diabetes

People newly diagnosed with Type 1 diabetes in the UK will almost invariably receive their initial education and management through secondary care. A new approach to weight management, food intake and insulin dose adjustment is being trialled in the UK at present. This Dose Adjustment For Normal Eating (DAFNE) programme involves a structured training course in intensive insulin therapy and self-management, which takes place on an outpatient basis.[12] People with Type 1 diabetes are taught to match their insulin dose to food intake on a meal-by-meal basis. The aim is to enable people to maintain healthy glycaemic control without an increased risk of severe hypoglycaemia and with minimal support from health care professionals. The study has shown improved control without more hypoglycaemic episodes, improved quality of life and satisfaction with treatment.

Case history

Mrs MS was a 73-year-old lady with a BMI of 33, who presented to her GP with symptoms of tiredness and lethargy. On direct questioning she admitted to thirst and polyuria, but didn't feel acutely ill. Blood tests were normal apart from a blood glucose level of 42 mmol! A diagnosis of diabetes was made.

She said she had been drinking at least four cups of tea per day, and was putting three teaspoons of sugar in each one. She was also drinking a least two litres of lemonade per day. She changed to using artificial sweeteners and sugar-free lemonade, and was closely monitored. She was encouraged to lose weight and exercise. Over the next two months her blood glucose levels slowly normalised. After one year her HbA1c was 7.2% on diet and exercise only, and her BMI had dropped to 29.

Actions for primary care

1. Weigh people at each diabetes clinic visit, and calculate BMI.
2. Encourage people with Type 2 diabetes in healthy eating and physical activity so that they can optimise their weight. A BMI of around 25 is ideal.
3. Try to set up group education sessions.
4. Consider referring people with Type 1 diabetes to a DAFNE programme if this might be of benefit to them.

Summary points

• Weight management is the cornerstone of treatment in Type 2 diabetes.
• Modest weight loss in the overweight person can help to delay or prevent the onset of diabetes.

- Education – especially for healthy eating – is a vital part of diabetes management.
- Weighing at each clinic visit is vital. Clinical computer systems will then automatically calculate BMI.

References

1. Gadsby R. Epidemiology of diabetes. *Advanced Drug Delivery Reviews* 2002; **54**: 1165–72
2. Tuomilehto J, Lindstrom MS, Eriksson JG *et al*. Prevention of type 2 diabetes mellitus by changes in lifestyle among subjects with impaired glucose tolerance. *N Engl J Med* 2001; **344**: 1343–9
3. Diabetes Prevention Programme Research Group. Reduction in the incidence of Type 2 diabetes with lifestyle intervention or metformin. *N Engl J Med* 2002; **346**: 393–403
4. Torgerson JS, Hauptman J, Boldrin M, Sjostrom L. XENical in the prevention of diabetes in obese subjects (XENDOS) study. *Diabetes Care* 2004; **27**: 155–61
5. Scottish Intercollegiate Guidelines Network. *Management of Diabetes: SIGN guideline 55*. Edinburgh: SIGN, Nov 2001 www.sign.ac.uk/guidelines/fulltext/55/index.html (accessed 30 Sept 2004)
6. United Kingdom Prospective Diabetes Study Group (UKPDS). Response of fasting glucose to diet therapy in newly presenting Type 2 diabetic patients (UKPDS 7). *Metabolism* 1990; **39**: 905–12
7. NICE. *Guidance on the use of patient-education models for diabetes. Technology appraisal 60*. London: NICE, April 2003 www.nice.org.uk/pdf/60Patienteducationmodelsfullguidance.pdf (accessed 28 Sept 2004)
8. Kinmonth AL, Woodcock A, Griffin S, Spiegal N, Campbell MJ. Randomised controlled trial of patient-centred care of diabetes in general practice: impact on current wellbeing and future disease risk. *BMJ* 1998; **317(7167)**: 1202–8
9. Department of Health. *National Service Framework for Diabetes: Standards*. London: HMSO, 2001 www.dh.gov.uk/assetRoot/04/05/89/38/04058938.pdf (accessed 28 Sept 2004)
10. International Diabetes Federation. *International Consensus Standards of Practice for Diabetes Education*. London: IDF Diabetes Education Consultative Section (DECS), 1997. www.idf.org/webdata/docs/International%20standards.pdf (accessed 28 Sept 2004)
11. Survival kit: the five-minute education kit. A document for health care providers and patients. Diabetes education study group of the European Association for the Study of Diabetes. *Diabet Med* 1995; **12**: 1022–43
12. DAFNE Study Group. Training in flexible, intensive insulin management to enable dietary freedom with Type 1 diabetes; dose adjustment for normal eating (DAFNE) randomised controlled trial. *BMJ* 2002; **325**: 746–9

SMOKING

Diabetes quality indicator 3 (DM3)

The percentage of patients with diabetes in whom there is a record of smoking status in the previous 15 months except those who have never smoked where smoking status should be recorded once.

Minimum threshold = 25%, maximum threshold to earn full available 3 points = 90%

Diabetes quality indicator 4 (DM4)

The percentage of patients who smoke whose notes contain that smoking cessation advice has been offered in the past 15 months.

Minimum threshold = 25%, maximum to earn full available 3 points = 90%

Background

The prevalence of smoking appears to be essentially the same for individuals with and without diabetes.[1] In the UK, at present, 27% of the population continue to smoke. Smoking cessation decreases the risk of coronary heart disease, cancer, stroke, and lung disease.[2] People with diabetes may also be able to reduce their risk of some diabetes microvascular complications by quitting smoking.[3]

Evidence base from trials

There is substantial evidence from patient series, case-control and cohort studies that smoking in people with diabetes is associated with both the development and progression of heart disease and nephropathy, and with the development of neuropathy. The evidence for an association with retinopathy is inconsistent. Smoking also increases the overall mortality in individuals with diabetes.[3]

There are no randomised controlled trials of smoking cessation specifically in people with diabetes. Evidence from studies in people who do not have diabetes suggests that smoking cessation will be associated with a significant reduction in risk of cardiovascular disease and death. Given that people with diabetes are already at increased risk of cardiovascular disease and diabetes microvascular complications, even a small decrease in their risk would be clinically meaningful.[3]

Recommendations from guidelines

Diabetes National Service Framework (NSF)

Smoking cessation in people with diabetes who smoke reduces their risk of both cardiovascular disease and microvascular complications (Level 2 evidence).[4]

Scottish Intercollegiate Guidelines Network (SIGN 55)

Health care professionals involved in caring for people with diabetes should advise them not to smoke (Level A recommendation).[5]

American Diabetes Association (ADA)

Prevention or cessation of tobacco use is an important component of diabetes clinical care.[6]

Effects of smoking cessation advice

Doctors have an important role to play in helping smokers to quit. Giving clear and simple advice to patients can increase the proportion of smokers who quit long term by 2–3%.[7] Results of various interventions are outlined in Table 5.1.[8]

Table 5.1 Effects of interventions in smoking cessation

Intervention	Abstinence rates at one year
Serious unaided attempt to quit	1–2%
Brief advice	3–5%
Brief advice plus leaflet	5–8%
Nicotine replacement therapy/ bupropion plus behaviour support	17%

There is a small amount of evidence that the results in Table 5.1, which were obtained in studies of people who did not have diabetes, may not be quite as high in populations who all have diabetes. Factors potentially inhibiting success in people with diabetes include fear of weight gain, depression and the use of smoking to suppress stress and anxiety related to diabetes management.[3] This may be particularly prevalent in smokers with Type 1 diabetes.[9]

Standard models for measuring stages of change (pre-contemplative, contemplative, preparation, action, maintenance and relapse) have been used to assess readiness to quit smoking. There is some evidence that interventions aimed at discussing the benefits of quitting smoking may be most useful for pre-contemplators and contemplators, whereas interventions aimed at promoting self-efficacy may be more useful for those preparing to quit. The SIGN guidelines suggest that a model using stages of change may help health care professionals understand how ready an individual is to quit smoking.

Pharmacological therapy

Nicotine replacement therapy (NRT) is effective in increasing the rate of quitting. All the forms of NRT – gum, patch, nasal spray, inhaler and sublingual tablets – have broadly similar efficacy.[3] There is no evidence of benefit of NRT in those smoking less than 15 cigarettes a day. Highly dependent smokers may benefit from more NRT and may need a higher dose. Eight weeks of patch therapy has been shown to be as effective as a longer duration of therapy.

The SIGN guidelines recommend that NRT should be provided for smokers of more than 15 cigarettes a day who are trying to quit. Therapy in a form acceptable to the patient should be offered for up to eight weeks.[3]

Bupropion increases the rate of smoking cessation.[3] A combination of this agent with NRT is more efficacious than using a patch alone. However, these studies were not carried out specifically in people with diabetes. The summary of product characteristics recommends a lower dose of bupropion in patients on oral hypoglycaemic agents or insulin, as there is a greater risk of seizure.

The SIGN guidelines recommend that bupropion therapy (in the absence of contraindications) could be used alone or in combination with NRT if blood pressure is monitored.[3]

Case history

Mr KH was a 47-year-old man who had smoked 20 cigarettes per day for 30 years. His BMI was 27 and he had just been diagnosed with diabetes. He had a manual job and was eating a healthy diet. Smoking cessation was discussed at his practice diabetes clinic appointment and he decided he wanted to give up. He was referred to the practice nurse-led smoking cessation clinic. He received support, follow up and a course of nicotine replacement therapy. A year later he was not smoking, but his BMI had risen to 29!

Actions for primary care

1. Enquire about smoking status at each visit to the practice diabetes service and record this on the clinical computer system template. This should use the codes: 137i never smoked, 137L ex-smoker, 137R smoker.
2. Set up a practice 'Stop Smoking Service' by ensuring that the practice nurse has the education, support materials, protocols and training to run this.
3. Offer smoking cessation advice to all people with diabetes who smoke, and record this on the practice clinical computer system using the 8CAL Read code.
4. Refer them to the practice 'Stop Smoking Service'.

> **Summary points**
> - Health care professionals should advise all people who have diabetes and who smoke to quit, and record this on the diabetes template.
> - Practices should run a 'Stop Smoking Service' to support people to stop smoking.

References

1. Haire-Joshu D, Glasgow RE, Tibbs TL. Smoking and Diabetes (Technical review). *Diabetes Care* 1999; **22**: 1887–98
2. Department of Health. *Smoking Kills. A White Paper on Tobacco.* London: HMSO, 1998
3. Wingard D, Barrett-Connor E, Wedick N. What is the evidence that changing tobacco use reduces the incidence of diabetic complications. In: Williams R, Herman W, Kinmonth A-L, Wareham N (eds). *The Evidence Base for Diabetes Care*, Chichester: Wiley Publishers, 2002, Ch.19
4. Department of Health. *National Service Framework for Diabetes: Standards.* London: HMSO, 2001 www.dh.gov.uk/assetRoot/04/05/89/38/04058938.pdf (accessed 28 Sept 2004)
5. Scottish Intercollegiate Guidelines Network. *Management of Diabetes: SIGN guideline 55.* Edinburgh: SIGN, Nov 2001 www.sign.ac.uk/guidelines/fulltext/55/index.html (accessed 30 Sept 2004)
6. American Diabetes Association. Smoking and Diabetes (Position Statement). *Diabetes Care* 2000; **23**: 93–4
7. Law M, Tang J. An analysis of the effectiveness of interventions intended to help people stop smoking. *Arch Int Med* 1995; **155**: 1933–41
8. Gregory S, Bason S. Smoking Cessation: is it worth the effort? Update 6 March 2003
9. Haire-Joshu D, Heady S, Thomas L *et al.* Beliefs about smoking and diabetes care. *Diabetes Educ* 1994; **20(5)**: 410–15

Diabetes quality indicator 5 (DM5)

The percentage of diabetic patients who have a record of HbA1c or equivalent in the previous 15 months:

Minimum threshold = 25%, maximum threshold to learn full three available points = 90%

Diabetes quality indicator 6 (DM6)

The percentage of patients with diabetes in whom the last HbA1c is 7.4% or less (or equivalent test/reference range depending on local laboratory) in last 15 months:

Minimum threshold = 25%, maximum threshold to learn full 16 available points = 50%

Diabetes quality indicator 7 (DM7)

The percentage of patients with diabetes in whom the last HbA1c is 10% or less (or equivalent test/reference range depending on local laboratory) in last 15 months:

Minimum threshold = 25%, maximum threshold to learn full 11 available points = 85%

Background

The three points for HbA1c process and the 27 points for HbA1c quality, indicate the importance of good glycaemic control in quality diabetes management. There is a good evidence base to show the value of good glycaemic control as measured by HbA1c, in the prevention of complications in diabetes.

Evidence base for good glycaemic control

There is high-quality evidence from randomised controlled trials in both Type 1 and Type 2 diabetes, that intensive control of blood glucose (giving HbA1c measurements of 7% or less), reduces the risk of adverse outcomes.

Type 1 diabetes

In the Diabetes Control and Complications Trial (DCCT) 1441 people with Type 1 diabetes aged between 16 and 39 years, were divided into two groups. One group was intensively controlled and had HbA1c measurements averaging 7%, the other group received standard care and had HbA1c levels averaging 9%. They were monitored for an average of 6.5 years.

Findings showed that intensive treatment reduced the risk of severe retinopathy by 47% and the need for laser treatment by 56%. It also reduced the risk of developing microalbuminuria by 54% and the risk of neuropathy by 60%.[1]

The groups were followed up after the trial finished. Once the intensive support in the trial ended, the glycaemic control in the intensive group deteriorated to an average HbA1c of 8%. However, the glycaemic control in the standard treatment group improved to 8%. The groups continued to be followed and a paper was published with results of a further six years follow-up showing that the group who were intensively treated continued to have less complications and less carotid intima-media thickness which is a marker for atherosclerosis.[2] The conclusion is that intensive control, even for a limited time, has long-term benefits in reducing microvascular complications and carotid intima-media thickness, a surrogate marker for macrovascular complications.

Type 2 diabetes

In the United Kingdom Prospective Diabetes Study (UKPDS) 5102 people with newly-diagnosed Type 2 diabetes initially underwent three months' diet treatment. Then, 4209 of these who were asymptomatic and had fasting plasma glucose levels between 6 and 15 mmol/l were randomised into an intensively treated group – who had an average HbA1c of 7.9% – and a conventionally treated group, who had an average HbA1c of 7%.

Follow-up was on average for 10 years. The intensive group had 12% less risk of any diabetes-related adverse endpoint, 25% fewer adverse microvascular endpoints and 16% fewer myocardial infarctions (this figure for major macrovascular outcomes did not reach statistical significance).[3] Neither sulphonylurea or insulin therapy showed any advantage over each other, but a group of obese patients randomised to metformin had substantially better macrovascular outcomes.[4]

These UKPDS glycaemic data have also been published in an epidemiological form in which it can be shown that adverse outcomes are lessened for any reduction in HbA1c level even if a target of 7% is not reached, thus a reduction of HbA1c from 10% to 9% is of benefit.[5]

Recommendations from guidelines on HbA1c targets

The Scottish SIGN guidelines

These recommend that good glycaemic control (HbA1C around 7%) should be maintained in all patients with diabetes.[6]

The NICE guidelines on management of Type 2 diabetes

For glucose control NICE recommends HbA1c be kept in the range 6.5–7.5% to minimise adverse outcomes.[7]

Box 6.1 Tools to achieve good glycaemic control in Type 2 diabetes

---

- Nutrition and exercise therapy
  This is covered in chapter four.
- Oral agents
  Once nutrition and exercise alone is insufficient to achieve good glycaemic control oral agents need to be introduced. Several groups are available.

Insulin secretagoges (sulphonylureas and short-acting secretagoges)

What are they?

There are six sulphonylureas available in the UK, glimepiride, glibenclamide, gliclazide, glipizide, gliquidone and tolbutamide. There are two short-acting insulin secretagoges, repaglinide and netaglinide.

How do they work?

They stimulate insulin release from the pancreatic B-cell, and are therefore dependent on the patient having adequate B-cell function. The main difference between members of the group is duration of action. Tolbutamide needs to be given three times per day, whilst the action of glibenclamide may last more than 24 hours. The short-acting secretagoges work within 10–30 mins of ingestion and have a duration of action from two to four hours. They are given with each meal.

How well do they work?

They reduce glucose levels in monotherapy or in combination with metformin effectively and usually within a few days, giving HbA1c reductions of around 1 to 1.5%.

Who should have them?

They can be used as monotherapy if diet alone is insufficient, in thin people, and in those who have symptomatic hyperglycaemia when their rapid onset of action can be helpful in reducing symptoms quickly. They can be used with metformin in dual therapy. The short-acting agent repaglinide can be used in monotherapy or with metformin. Netaglinide can only be used with metformin. These short-acting agents are used with each meal, so they are useful if people have erratic eating patterns, for example, shift workers.

Do they have any side effects?

Hypoglycaemia is the main one. This is more likely to occur with glibenclamide, because of its long half-life. They are usually well-tolerated but most can cause weight gain.

Who should avoid having them?

Glibenclamide-induced hypoglycaemia has been described mainly in older people and those with neurological impairment. It is advised not to begin therapy with glibenclamide in people over 70 years of age.

They should also be avoided in people with severe renal and liver impairment.

Biguanides

What are they?

Metformin is the only biguanide available in the UK.

How does it work?

Metformin inhibits hepatic glucose production and enhances insulin-stimulated glucose uptake and glycogenesis by skeletal muscle. It improves some of the metabolic actions of insulin and has additional beneficial effects independent of insulin. It does not stimulate insulin production.

How well does it work?

It lowers HbA1c in line with all other oral agents, lowering HbA1c by 1–2%. In the UKPDS study metformin had benefits over and above its glycaemic lowering effects of reducing adverse macrovascular outcomes, and so it is recommended as the initial monotherapy of choice in overweight people with diabetes.

Does it have any side effects?

Metformin is excreted in the urine. The rare serious side effect associated with metformin is lactic acidosis, and this can happen if metformin accumulates in the body where there is renal impairment. Guidelines therefore suggest stopping metformin if the serum creatinine level rises above 150 mmol/l.

Metformin can give rise to gastrointestinal side effects of abdominal pain, nausea, diarrhoea and a metallic taste in the mouth. Around 10–20% do not continue on metformin because of these side effects. They can be minimised by starting with a low dose say 500mgs daily and titrating up to 500mgs twice daily over two to four weeks.

Who should avoid metformin?

Because of the risk of lactic acidosis, metformin is contraindicated in people with uncontrolled heart failure, renal failure and advanced liver disease.

Thiazolidinediones

What are they?

Two thiazolidinediones, or glitazones as they are more easily called, are available in the UK. They are pioglitazone and rosiglitazone.

How do they work?

They work mainly by stimulating a nuclear receptor called peroxisome proliferator-activated receptor-gamma (PPARy), which is most strongly expressed in adipose tissue. It acts to increase transcription of certain insulin-sensitive genes involved in the control of lipid and glucose metabolism – as a result, they lower insulin resistance.

How well do they work?

Glitazones produce a slowly generated blood glucose lowering effect in Type 2 diabetes that may take from three to six months to achieve maximal effect. In combination treatment with metformin, glitazones lower HbA1c in the range 0.6–1.2%.

Who should have them?

The licence indications in the UK are at present quite restricted. They state that glitazones can be used in oral combination therapy for patients with insufficient glycaemic control, despite maximal tolerated dose of oral monotherapy with either metformin or a sulphonylurea:

- in combination with metformin only in obese patients
- in combination with a sulphonylurea only in patients who show intolerance to metformin or in whom it is contraindicated
- as oral monotherapy in people who are intolerant to metformin or in whom metformin is contraindicated.

Do they have any side effects?

Glitazones are generally well-tolerated. The main side effect is fluid retention with increased plasma volume, reduced haematocrit, and a decrease in haemoglobin. As a result peripheral oedema, mainly at the ankles, may occur in some patients. There may be an associated weight gain of around 5%.

A previously released glitazone called troglitazone was withdrawn due to cases of fatal hepatotoxicity. Pioglitazone and rosiglitazone have been used extensively in the USA and none of the liver toxicity found with troglitazone has been reported. However, the licence specifies that liver function tests are to be undertaken before therapy, every two months for the first year and at appropriate intervals thereafter.

Who should avoid having them?

The current licence states that they should not be used with insulin. They should also not be used where there is a history of heart failure, liver impairment or severe kidney problems.

Other notes

A combination tablet of metformin and rosiglitazone is now available in the UK.

Alpha-glucosidase inhibitors (acarbose)

What are they?

The only agent that is available in the UK is acarbose.

How does it work?

Acarbose reduces the rise in blood glucose that occurs after a meal by inhibiting the enzyme, alpha glucosidase, which breaks down carbohydrates into monosaccharides in the small intestine. As a result carbohydrates pass further down into the large bowel.

How well does it work?

It can reduce HbA1c between 0.6–1%.

Who should have it?

It can be used as monotherapy, in any combination with any other agent or agents, and with insulin.

Does it have any side effects?

The extra carbohydrate that gets into the large bowel is digested by bowel micro-organisms producing flatulence, bloating and diarrhoea. To try to minimise these side effects the drug should be started at low dose and titrated up. Begin with a 50mg tablet with one meal each day for two weeks, then increase to one 50mg tablet with each of two meals a day for two weeks, then one 50mg tablet three times daily, increasing to a maximum of 100mg three times daily. These side effects severely limit its use amongst people in the UK, and the drug is no longer promoted in the UK.

Who should avoid taking it?

Anyone who continues to eat a high carbohydrate diet.

Using oral agents to keep HbA1c to target in Type 2 diabetes

In people who are overweight, defined as BMI over 25 in Caucasian people, or above 23 in Indo-Asian people:

Step one

- Begin metformin at 500mg daily, titrate up over two to four weeks to 500mg twice daily, increasing to 1g twice daily as necessary.

  If not tolerated consider sulphonylurea or glitazone.

Rationale

The NICE guidelines on glycaemic control in Type 2 diabetes recommend that metformin be the initial monotherapy of choice in all people who are overweight, defined as a BMI greater than 25. It also states that metformin should be considered as initial monotherapy in those with a BMI under 25.

This is because it is felt that metformin has the added value of reducing cardiovascular events in addition to its effect on blood glucose lowering. This view comes from data from the UKPDS research study.

It has been suggested that this benefit may come partly because metformin works by affecting the way that insulin is utilised in the body, rather than by stimulating the pancreas to release more insulin, which is the mechanism of action of the sulphonylurea group of drugs.

Metformin, however, causes side effects in a number of people. This can mean that up to 20% of people may find it impossible to take metformin.

If someone is unable to take metformin should they be offered a sulphonylurea or a glitazone as their initial monotherapy? Those favouring the sulphonylurea approach might say that they are well-known drugs that have few side effects or contraindications. They reliably and quickly reduce blood glucose levels, and are therefore particularly helpful if the person has symptoms attributable to hyperglycaemia. They are also relatively cheap. The problem is that they may cause weight gain and, in contrast to metformin, they do not reduce adverse cardiovascular events.

Those favouring the glitazone route argue that by using a drug that is treating the underlying condition of insulin resistance, they are dealing with one of the main causes of Type 2 diabetes. The best clinical marker of insulin resistance is obesity, and so the use of a glitazone in obese individuals is particularly appropriate. They argue the use of a sulphonylurea will only stimulate more insulin release in a person who is insulin resistant, so that the hyperglycaemic effect may be blunted, and the risks of weight gain increased.

In people who have BMI under 25 (or 23 if Indo-Asian), especially if they have symptoms of hyperglycaemia, e.g. thirst, tiredness, and weight loss:

Step one

- Consider metformin, but if considered inappropriate, begin on sulphonylurea of choice at low dose, and titrate up.

Rationale

Metformin takes several weeks to achieve significant reductions in symptoms, whereas sulphonylureas work quickly. Remember that the thin person presenting with many diabetes symptoms may have Type 1 diabetes. Keep a close watch on such people, see them every few weeks and monitor the effects of therapy by measuring fasting glucose levels. Titrate the dose of sulphonylurea up until the fasting glucose is controlled. If maximum doses fail to control glycaemia, introduce insulin therapy quickly.

If oral monotherapy with metformin at maximum tolerated dose does not reduce HbA1c to target:

Step two
- Add sulphonylurea (or glitazone) – see rationale above. Titrate dose of second agent up to maximum tolerated dose.

If therapy with two agents at maximum tolerated doses does not reduce HbA1c to target:

Step three
- Consider adding once-daily insulin or add acarbose or consider triple therapy with metformin/sulphonylurea/ glitazone.

Rationale
The addition of acarbose is only likely to yield a reduction in HbA1c of less than 1% and many will not tolerate its side effects. Some people will easily accept that they need insulin and be prepared to try it. Others, either because of their jobs or through fear of injections, will not want to consider insulin.

Triple therapy with metformin/sulphonylurea/glitazone represents off-licence prescribing for the glitazone, but is becoming quite widely used.[8] Once this line of management has been discussed and agreed with the person with diabetes, consent should be recorded in the notes.

Deciding that this person would benefit from insulin
There is no strong evidence base to determine exactly when insulin therapy should be introduced, but it should be considered in patients who meet the following criteria:
- poor glycaemic control as evidenced by persistently elevated HbA1c (no consensus as to exactly what level, but above the 7.4% target)

- symptoms of polyuria, polydipsia, nocturia and/or recurrent infections such as balanitis and thrush
- currently receiving maximal dosage of oral agents
- has already optimised lifestyle changes.

A key factor that will need to be addressed is the individual's views, attitudes and fears. These usually involve worries about the fear and pain of injections, and the risks of hypoglycaemia. The needles used for insulin injections today are very short and thin, and as a result injections are almost pain-free. The risks of hypoglycaemia may be minimised by using simple insulin regimes, continuing oral agent therapy with metformin, and considering using once-daily insulin glargine with its lower hypoglycaemic risk profile.

Controlling glycaemia in people with Type 1 diabetes

Most people in the UK with Type 1 diabetes will have received their initial education and management in secondary care. Many will still be attending secondary care diabetes clinics for their diabetes management. Some however, for whatever reason, will no longer be under hospital care. Many will know much about their diabetes and will be adept at varying their insulin dose, and will have clear ideas about the level of HbA1c they wish to try to attain. Some, however, will want encouragement and help to achieve their HbA1c target. This will usually require a discussion of food intake, the level of physical activity being undertaken, and insulin dose adjustment.

In order to advise on insulin dose adjustment for people with Type 1 and Type 2 diabetes – and to be able to start people with Type 2 diabetes on insulin – information about insulins, insulin delivery systems and insulin regimes is needed.

Types of insulin

The large majority of people today use human-sequence insulin. It is manufactured using recombinant DNA technology in which the human insulin genes are inserted into yeast or bacteria cells which can be grown in bulk and the human insulin harvested from the cells. Pork and beef insulin, extracted and purified from animal pancreases is still available for those who need it.

Short- and longer-acting forms of insulin exist:

Short-acting insulins

These are known as clear, or soluble, insulins. They have a peak action from two to six hours after injection. They should be given from 20 to 30 mins before meals. One of the best known examples is Human Actrapid.

Longer-acting insulins

These are cloudy insulins. They are made by precipitating insulin or protamine-insulin in the presence of zinc. This forms insoluble crystals that are injected as a suspension and absorbed slowly. These insulins have a peak action at around eight hours after injection, but their effect may last for up to 18 hours in some people.

Pre-mixed insulins

These contain combinations of soluble, short-acting and crystalline long-acting insulin. A combination of 30% short-acting and 70% long-acting is one that is often used, but 10:90, 15:85, 20:80, 25:75, 40:60, and 50:50 combinations are produced by different companies.

Short-acting insulin analogues

These have been developed by minor alterations to the amino acid sequences of human insulin to produce insulins that have a quicker onset of action, and shorter duration of action than normal soluble insulin. Two are available, insulin lispro – which is identical to human insulin apart from inversion of lysine and proline residues at positions B28 and B29 on the B chain of the insulin molecule, and insulin aspart – which is identical to human insulin apart from the substitution of proline at position B28 with aspartic acid.

Both analogues have similar pharmacokinetic profiles, peak action is around one hour after injection and their effect wanes after four hours. This means that they can be injected just before a meal and they reduce the risk of postprandial hypoglycaemia.

They are now available pre-mixed with longer-acting cloudy insulins in varying combinations for those using a twice daily pre-mix regime.

Long-acting insulin analogue

Insulin glargine is the first long-acting analogue to be developed and marketed. It is the same as human insulin apart from a substitution of glycine for asparagine on the A chain of the insulin molecule at position A21 and the addition of two arginine molecules at the C-terminal end of the B chain. This results in a change in properties of insulin glargine. It is soluble at acidic pH and so is the first clear, long-acting insulin. When it is injected it forms a microprecipitate within the more neutral pH of the subcutaneous tissues. This results in slow absorption from the injection site. It has a flat profile of action with no pronounced peaks, a duration of action of around 24 hours and is subject to less inter- and intra-person variability than previous cloudy long-acting insulins.[9] As a result, there is often a reduction in hypoglycaemic episodes in people using insulin glargine.

Another long-acting insulin analogue, insulin detemir, has recently been launched in the UK. It is a modified human insulin with a 14-carbon fatty-acid chain attached at position B29 of the insulin amino acid sequence and the amino acid threonine at position B30 removed. It is a soluble formulation and remains in solution after injection. The mechanism by which insulin detemir protracts action is a combination of increased self-association and albumin binding. Evidence from studies shows that glycaemic control is more predictable with detemir than with traditional long-acting isophane insulin and with less nocturnal hypoglycaemia.[10]

Insulin delivery systems

Most insulins are available in 10 ml vials, pen cartridges and disposable pens. A good analogy is that of pen and writing. Vials are like dipping a quill into ink, insulin cartridges are like cartridge pens, and disposable pens are biros! Pen technology enables insulin to be carried about easily and enables injections to be given where and when required. Insulin doses can be dialled-up more accurately using the pen devices, and it is easier to teach people to use pen devices than it is to draw up insulin into a syringe from a vial. Most people moving on to insulin when offered a choice prefer pen devices and they are now commonly being prescribed for initiation of insulin in both Type 1 and Type 2 diabetes. Some health care professionals prefer cartridges and others the disposable pens. Patient choice should inform the decision as to which to use.

A few people with Type 1 diabetes use continuous infusion pumps, which give a slow steady infusion of short-acting insulin. Pump technology has developed significantly in the past few years. However, it is expensive and there are limited NHS funds for it. People using this will be under the care of a secondary or tertiary diabetes care centre.

Insulin regimes

Basal–bolus therapy is the insulin regime in which an injection of short-acting insulin is given just before each meal with one injection of long-acting insulin at night. People using this regime usually have four injections per day. It allows the flexibility to cope with different meal times, size of meals and exercise.

Another regime is to have two daily injections of pre-mixed insulin, one before breakfast and the other before the evening meal.

Getting HbA1c to target level in Type 1 diabetes

- Discuss eating habits, food intake, physical activity and any hypoglycaemic episodes.
- Adjust insulin dose upwards, depending on overall HbA1c level, and home blood glucose monitoring results.

  If the person is on a twice-daily mixed insulin regime discuss changing to a basal–bolus regime, which gives greater flexibility, and a greater chance of achieving the HbA1c target.

  If the person is on a basal–bolus regime but is poorly controlled or is having hypoglycaemic episodes consider changing to a basal–bolus regime using short-acting analogue insulins with meals and the long-acting analogue insulin, insulin glargine, once daily.

Starting someone with Type 2 diabetes on insulin

People with Type 2 diabetes who come to need insulin may be best controlled on one injection of long-acting insulin per day, with the continuation of some or all of their oral agents.[9]

Before start of insulin

- teach home blood glucose monitoring if not already doing it
- revise and reinforce dietary principles

Initiation of insulin

- stop glitazone but continue on metformin at 1g bd (if tolerated) and sulphonylurea
- teach insulin injection technique
- define initial dose of insulin (long-acting analogue or NPH), one injection in the evening
- safe starting dose = fasting glucose level as units of insulin, i.e. if fasting glucose is 10, starting dose is 10 units
- give verbal and written instructions about increasing glucose dose by two units if three consecutive fasting blood glucose are above 5.5 mmol

- teach about hypoglycaemia symptoms and treatment
- give contact telephone number for advice and help

Follow up

- by phone after a couple of days and then individualise frequency of calls depending on progress, need to alter insulin dose, and blood glucose control
- HbA1c every three months until stabilised

    The techniques of how to dial-up the correct dose of insulin from a pen device, giving the injection and adjustment of insulin dosage all need to be demonstrated, and taught. The person newly starting on insulin needs to be observed giving an injection. They then need close support and supervision over the first few days and weeks. Diabetes specialist nurses (DSNs) are the health care professionals that have traditionally done this work. Practice nurses in some areas are beginning to initiate insulin with the support of GPs, local DSNs and consultant diabetologists. There are now short courses available on insulin initiation in primary care to teach these skills.

    In some areas, groups of individuals are being initiated on insulin in so-called 'group start' programmes often supervised by a DSN working in the community. Insulin initiation in Type 2 diabetes is moving from the secondary care/DSN environment to the primary care/ practice nurse environment. This will enable more people to be treated to the HbA1c quality target of 7.4%.

Exception reporting for glycaemia

It may be impossible or undesirable for an individual to get to the 7.4% HbA1c target because of patient choice or significant co-morbidities. A Read code has been developed to allow such people to be excluded from the total numbers of people with diabetes from which the 50% at HbA1c of 7.4% or below are calculated. The code for maximum tolerated dose of hypoglycaemic medication is 8BL0.00, the code for patient unsuitable is 9h41.09.

Case history

> Mr B is 79 and has Type 2 diabetes and severe demen-
> tia. He is on maximum tolerated doses of oral agents
> and an HbA1c of 9%. He lives in a care home. He can-
> not exercise because of osteoarthritis, and his BMI and
> diet are ideal.
>
> The next step in pharmacotherapy would be the ad-
> dition of insulin. However, for Mr B this could add such
> a risk of hypoglycaemia as to make it medically unsafe
> to suggest insulin.

Case history

> Mrs H is 37 and has had Type 1 diabetes for 21 years.
> She has had problems with hypoglycaemic episodes for
> many years and has become very frightened of them.
> She is well-informed about her diabetes and decides
> that she wishes to keep her HbA1c in the range 7.5%–
> 8% in order to minimise the risk of hypoglycaemia.

Other situations where exception reporting will be
needed are for people with terminal illness, and in people who have just been diagnosed or who have just registered with the practice, when three months' grace is
allowed in order to collect the data and optimise glycaemic control.

Relevance of glycaemic targets in the elderly

The UKPDS study recruited newly-diagnosed people
with diabetes up to the age of 65 and followed them for
a mean of 12.7 years. This suggests that there can be an
evidence base for tight glycaemic control for people up
to their late 70s. However there are no glycaemic control
studies that have been performed specifically in populations over the age of 75 years.

It can be suggested that people who are in their late
70s or early 80s and who have a single disease model
should aim for an HbA1c at or below the 7.4% target. Patients in this category have no evidence of other serious

co-morbidities, no cognitive impairment, and are generally self-caring. Unfortunately, only about one third of elderly subjects fall into this category, according to the results of a large community-based sample of people with diabetes over the age of 65 years.[11]

The other two thirds, because of frailty and other co-morbidities, may not benefit from trying to reach the 7.4% HbA1c target. After discussion and individualised glycaemic target setting, a higher level of HbA1c target may be considered appropriate, and the person excluded from data collection using the exception code.

Action points for primary care
1. Use exclusion codes to rule out those for whom tight glycaemic control is inappropriate.
2. Measure HbA1c at least annually.
3. Encourage people with Type 2 diabetes to have good diabetes control by reinforcing lifestyle change, titrating up doses of oral agents, adding new agents or starting insulin as appropriate.
4. Encourage people with Type 1 diabetes to achieve good control by reinforcing lifestyle advice, increasing insulin doses or altering insulin therapy as appropriate.

Summary points
- There is very good evidence in both Type 1 and Type 2 diabetes that good glycaemic control reduces adverse outcomes.
- Glycaemic control can be optimised by reinforcing lifestyle advice, and titrating therapy as appropriate.
- Exclusion codes can be used for those people in whom tight glycaemic control is inappropriate.

References
1. Diabetes Control and Complications Trial Research Group. The effect of intensive treatment on the development and progression of long term complications in insulin dependent diabetes mellitus. *N Engl J Med* 1993; **329:** 977–986
2. DCCT & Epidemiology of Diabetes Interventions and Complications

research group (EDIC). Intensive diabetes therapy and carotid intima-media thickness in type 1 diabetes. *N Engl J Med* 2003; **348(23):** 2294–303

3. United Kingdom Prospective Diabetes Study UKPDS 33. Intensive blood glucose control with sulphonylureas or insulin compared with conventional treatment and risk of complications in patients with Type 2 diabetes. *Lancet* 1998; **352:** 837–53

4. United Kingdom Prospective Diabetes Study UKPDS 34. Effect of intensive blood glucose control with metformin on complications in overweight patients with Type 2 diabetes. *Lancet* 1998; **352:** 854–65

5. United Kingdom Prospective Diabetes Study (UKPDS 35). Association of glycaemia with macrovascular and microvascular complications of Type 2 diabetes (UKPDS 35): prospective observational study BMJ 2000; **321:** 405–12

6. Scottish Intercollegiate Guidelines Network. *Management of Diabetes: SIGN guideline 55.* Edinburgh: SIGN, Nov 2001 www.sign.ac.uk/guidelines/fulltext/55/index.html (accessed 30 Sept 2004)

7. NICE Inherited Clinical Guideline G Management of Type 2 diabetes: management of blood glucose. London: NICE, Sept 2000

8. Byrne J, Garg S, Vaidya A, Rajbhandari SM, Wallis SC Efficacy of triple therapy with rosiglitazone, metformin and a sulphonylurea in lowering HbA1c. *Practical Diabetes International* 2003; **20:** 58–60

9. Gadsby R. Using insulin earlier in the treatment of type 2 diabetes. *British Journal of Diabetes and Vascular Disease* 2003; **3:** 119–22

10. Vague P, Selam J, Skeie S *et al.* Insulin detemir is associated with more predictable glycaemic control and reduced risk of hypoglycaemia compared to NPH insulin in subjects with type 1 diabetes on a basal–bolus regime with insulin as part. *Diabetes Care* 2003; **26(3):** 590–6

11. Sinclair AJ, Bayer AJ. All Wales Research in Elderly (AWARE) Diabetes Study, 121/3040. London: HMSO, 1998

7 RETINAL SCREENING

Diabetes quality indicator 8 (DM 8)
The percentage of patients with diabetes who have a record of retinal screening in the previous 15 months:
Minimum threshold = 25%, maximum threshold to earn full available 5 points = 90%

Background

Diabetic retinopathy is the leading cause of blindness in the UK in people of working age.[1] The pathophysiology is as yet incompletely understood, but it is thought that it involves damage to retinal blood vessels due to hyperglycaemia, leakage of plasma proteins through damaged blood vessels, and the proliferation of abnormal fragile blood vessels stimulated by the release of growth factors from the ischaemic retina.

The prevalence of retinopathy increases with the duration of diabetes and worsening of glycaemic control. In the Wisconsin epidemiological study of diabetic retinopathy, in those people with Type 2 diabetes, 20% had evidence of retinopathy within two years of diagnosis and 60% within 15 years of diagnosis.[2]

Many people who have diabetic retinopathy will be asymptomatic and have good vision. Even people with sight-threatening retinopathy may be asymptomatic. There is convincing evidence that regular surveillance for diabetic retinopathy in people with diabetes, and early laser treatment of those identified as having sight threatening retinopathy can reduce the incidence of new visual impairment and blindness.[3]

Therefore, the key issue is to identify those people with sight threatening retinopathy who will benefit from prophylactic treatment to prevent visual loss. A number of areas in the UK, over the past decade, have developed local retinal screening programmes based either on retinal photography or slit lamp bio-microscopy, usually performed by specially trained optometrists.

NSF target for retinal screening

The NSF for Diabetes: Delivery Strategy[4] gives very precise targets for retinal screening as follows:

By 2006, a minimum of 80% of people with diabetes are to be offered screening for the early detection (and treatment if needed) of diabetic retinopathy as part of a systematic programme that meets national standards, rising to 100% coverage of those at risk of retinopathy by the end of 2007.

Digital retinal photography or slit lamp bio-microscopy are the two modalities that achieve the sensitivity (80%) and specificity rates (95%) to make them acceptable for retinal screening.[5]

A National Retinopathy Screening Project Advisory Board has been set up following the Diabetes NSF Delivery Strategy document. A National Clinical Director for Diabetes has also been appointed. Together, they have said that the screening method to be used to achieve the NSF target will be digital retinal photography. Camera, service specifications, and outline costs for a district retinopathy screening programme based upon digital retinal photography are being published by the Advisory Committee. Mobile cameras will be needed to achieve the levels of coverage stated in the NSF, especially in rural populations. Optometrist-based schemes, and schemes based on photographic modalities other than digital imaging will need to be modified to conform to the new policy.

Classification of retinopathy and actions needed

The results of screening for diabetic retinopathy by digital photography carried out by the local programme will be sent back to general practitioners and will need to be put on the practice clinical computer system. There is now a nationally agreed classification of retinopathy, and actions that need to be taken as a result of screening.[6] These are shown in Table 7.1 below.

Table 7.1 Classification of retinopathy and action required

Grade	Features	Symptoms
Background	Microaneurysms Venous dilatation Scattered exudates Dot and blot haemorrhages	None
Preproliferative	Cotton wool spots Multiple haemorrhages Intra-retinal microvasular Abnormalities (IRMA) Venous beading, looping and duplication	None
Proliferative	New vessels on disc and elsewhere Fibrous proliferation on disc and elsewhere Preretinal and vitreous haemorrhages	None if uncomplicated but haemorrhage may give rise to visual loss
Advanced Diabetic Eye Disease	Retinal detachment and tears Extensive fibrovascular proliferation Vitreous haemorrhage Neovascular glaucoma	Visual loss or blindness
Maculopathy	Macular oedema Ischaemic maculopathy	Central visual loss

Actions to be taken – referral to an ophthalmology specialist

Table 7.2 How soon should patients be seen by the
ophthalmologist after referral

Same day	For sudden loss of vision and retinal detachment
Within one week	For new vessels, pre-retinal or vitreous haemorrhage Rubeosis iridis
Within four weeks	For unexplained drop in visual acuity, hard exudates within one disc diameter of fovea Macular oedema Pre-proliferative or severe retinopathy
Within three to six months	Worsening of lesions since previous screen Scattered exudates more than one disc diameter from fovea

Some screening programmes are developing direct referral guidelines so that the actions detailed above will
automatically be taken, and reported to the GP. In other
areas GPs still need to initiate these referrals. Specialist ophthalmology services need to be expanded to be
able to deliver the service standards outlined above. In
many areas there will need to be a rapid development
of laser clinic provision to provide treatment for people
with retinopathy.

Screening intervals

At present this is to be every year. There is some emerging evidence that those with no retinopathy at screening
are very unlikely to develop sight threatening retinopathy within three years. However, some people with background changes may progress to sight-threatening
retinopathy within a 12-month period.[7] It is possible,
therefore, that in the future those with no retinopathy
could be screened every two years and those with some
retinopathy might be screened every six to nine months.

Preparing people for screening

A call and recall system has to be set in place to ensure that people are invited to attend for retinal screening on a yearly basis. In some parts of the UK this is arranged as part of the retinal screening programme. In other areas screening invitations are generated and issued from individual general practices. People need to be made aware that their pupils will be dilated for the screening photograph and they should not therefore drive for about approximately four hours afterwards. Information leaflets that explain the screening process and give advice about being accompanied to the screening appointment are currently being produced.

Preparing people for laser treatment

When people are found to have retinopathy that requires referral and laser treatment they will need information about what laser treatment entails. Leaflets are being written to explain what is involved in laser treatment and these will hopefully be given out by the ophthalmology service.

Exclusion reporting

There are some people who, should they be found to have sight-threatening retinopathy, would be unsuitable for laser therapy. It would not therefore be ethical to screen them. These include those with terminal illness, and those with severe dementia and movement disorders. They should therefore be excluded. The Read code 9h41.09 indicates that a patient is unsuitable.

People who are registered blind are still offered screening by some programmes at present. This is because they may have a little useful vision, which could be protected by laser therapy. Partially-sighted people are included in the population to be screened.

Case history

Mr GH is a 76-year-old man who has had Type 2 diabetes for 15 years. At retinal screening he is found to have a dense right cataract and left proliferative retinopathy. His vision was 6/60 in his right eye and 6/9 in his left eye. He was referred to an ophthalmologist and was seen urgently. He needed to have an urgent right cataract extraction, as it was not possible to be clear about the degree of retinopathy behind it. This was carried out and he subsequently required laser treatment to both eyes. His vision two years later is 6/12 in both eyes.

Actions for primary care

1. Encourage all people with diabetes in the practice to attend for their annual retinopathy screening at the local retinopathy screening programme.
2. Provide information and advice about the screening.
3. Receive and record the results on the practice clinical computing system using the correct Read codes. Ensure that the appropriate actions on the results are taken.
4. Ensure that the local retinopathy screening programme is based on digital retinal photography of the required standard.
5. If this is based on a mobile camera, it may be that the camera-containing van will come to your practice car park on a yearly basis to do the screening. There then may be issues around the call and recall process for these people, and issues around who performs installation of eye drops for pupil dilatation that will need to be addressed.
6. Make sure that the local programme has developed a mechanism for screening those who are housebound and those in care homes.
7. Make sure that there are sufficient specialist ophthalmic and laser services provided locally to care for those found by screening.

Summary points

- There is good evidence that retinopathy screening of everyone with diabetes, and treatment with laser therapy of those found to have sight threatening retinopathy, will reduce blindness.
- It has been decided that digital retinal photography should be used as the screening modality in the UK.
- The NSF gives very definite targets of 80% screened by 2006 and 100% screened by end of 2007.
- General practice needs to receive and record the results of screening and ensure that appropriate action is taken.

References

1. Department of Health. *National Service Framework for Diabetes: Standards.* London: HMSO, 2001 www.dh.gov.uk/assetRoot/04/05/89/38/04058938.pdf (accessed 28 Sept 2004)
2. Klein R, Klein BEK, Moss SE *et al.* The Wisconsin Epidemiological Study of Diabetic Retinopathy 111. Prevalence and risk of diabetic retinopathy when age at diagnosis is 30 years or more. *Arch Ophthal* 1984; **102:** 527–32
3. Ferris F. Early photocoagulation in patients with either type 1 or type 2 diabetes. *Trans Am Ophthalmol Soc* 1996, **94:** 505–37
4. Department of Health. *National Service Framework for Diabetes: Delivery Strategy.* London: HMSO, December 2002 www.dh.gov.uk/assetRoot/04/03/28/23/04032823.pdf (accessed 28 Sept 2004)
5. Hutchinson A, McIntosh A, Peters J *et al.* Effectiveness of screening and monitoring tests for diabetic retinopathy – a systemic review. *Diabet Med* 2000; **17:** 495–506
6. Harding S, Greenwood R, Aldington S. Grading and disease management in national screening for diabetic retinopathy in England and Wales. *Diabet Med* 2003; **20:** 965–71
7. Kohner EM, Stratton IM, Aldington S *et al.* UK Prospective Diabetes Study (UKPDS) Group. Relationship between the severity of retinopathy and progression to photocoagulation in patients with Type 2 diabetes mellitus in the UKPDS (UKPDS 52). *Diabet Med* 2001; **18:** 178–84

8 FOOT CARE

Diabetes quality indicator 9 (DM9)
The percentage of patients with diabetes with a record of the presence or absence of peripheral pulses in the previous 15 months:
Minimum threshold = 25%, maximum threshold to earn full available 3 points = 90%

Diabetes quality indicator 10 (DM10)
The percentage of patients with diabetes with a record of neuropathy testing in the previous 15 months:
Minimum threshold = 25%, maximum threshold to earn full available 3 points = 90%

Background

Foot problems in diabetes result from complications such as peripheral vascular disease and neuropathy, which leads to loss of protective pain sensation in the feet. Between 20 and 40% of people with diabetes are estimated to have neuropathy depending on how it is defined and measured, and about 5% have a foot ulcer.[1] Foot ulcers may result in amputation. The incidence rate of diabetes-related lower limb amputation in one community study in the Tayside area of Scotland was 248 per 100,000 person years, which was 12.4 times higher than for the general population.[2]

Diabetic peripheral neuropathy is often asymptomatic, and the gradual loss of protective pain sensation usually isn't perceived by the person as it develops. Thus there are people with diabetes who have risk factors for foot ulceration and amputation of which they are not aware.

Approximately 50% of people with diabetes who attend dedicated foot clinics only have neuropathy. The other 50% have neuropathy plus some degree of reduced blood flow resulting from generalised atherosclerosis, which produces tissue ischaemia in the foot.[3]

Pure ischaemia without neuropathy is rare. Poor glycaemic control, duration of diabetes, and adverse socioeconomic conditions are other factors associated with increased risk of foot ulceration.

Feet that are at-risk due to neuropathy or ischaemia do not spontaneously ulcerate. Minor trauma is usually the additional factor that precipitates ulceration. The person with loss of protective pain sensation due to neuropathy may get trauma through thermal damage (e.g. walking on hot sand on holiday), chemical damage (e.g. use of corn-cures) or through mechanical trauma (e.g. tight-fitting shoes, standing on a stone or drawing pin). Foot ulcers are susceptible to infection which may spread rapidly causing overwhelming tissue destruction. This process is the main reason for amputation in people with diabetes who have neuropathy. The pathway to amputation is thus foot at risk, minor trauma, ulceration, spreading infection and amputation.

Potential strategies to reduce the risk of foot complications might include:

- early recognition of the at-risk foot
- appropriate regular clinical examination of the feet
- prompt referral for extra education
- intensive follow up for those with feet at-risk
- rapid referral for intensive treatment of foot ulcers in multidisciplinary foot clinics. [1,3]

Evidence-based recommendations for foot screening from NICE guidelines [1]

Regular (at least annual) visual inspection of the feet of the person with diabetes, assessment of foot sensation and palpation of foot pulses by trained personnel is important for the detection of risk factors for ulceration. *Recommendation grade A – based on category I evidence (see Table 2.1, chapter two).*

Examination of the feet should include:

- testing of foot sensation using a 10g nylon monofilament (see Figures 8.1a and b) or vibration

(using a biothesiometer, an electronic calibrated tuning fork)
- palpation of foot pulses (see Figures 8.2a and b)
- inspection of any foot deformity and footwear (recommendation grade A – based on category I evidence).

Monofilaments should not be used to test more than ten patients in any one session and should be left for 24 hours to recover (buckling strength) between sessions (recommendation grade C – based on category III evidence).

Classification of risk

People should be classified as at-risk if they have either inability to feel the 10g nylon monofilament and/or absent pulses and/or foot deformity. Those at risk need to be referred to the local foot at risk clinic run by the podiatry service to receive extra foot care education, further assessment to determine degree of risk, and appropriate follow up.[3]

Using the 10g nylon monofilament to detect neuropathy

The NICE report states that there is a good evidence base for the use of the biothesiometer and the 10g nylon monofilament to detect neuropathy.[1] The monofilament is easy to use, light and cheap compared with the biothesiometer, which often weighs 2.5kg, requires a power source and costs around £400.[4] The assessment of

Figure 8.1a and b
Using the 10g nylon microfilament to detect neuropathy

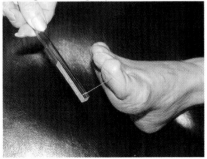 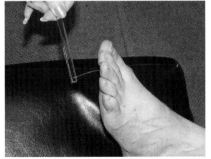

vibration using the 128 tuning fork is much less reliable as a test for neuropathy.

The NICE report states that identification of neuropathy, based on insensitivity to a 10g nylon monofilament is convenient and appears cost effective[1] (recommendation level grade C).

The filament is applied to at least five sites on the foot (but not over callus, which is an area of dry, hard, often fissured skin) until it buckles, which occurs at 10g of linear pressure when the patient is asked to detect its presence. If it cannot be felt, protective pain sensation is lost and neuropathy is present.

Diabetic peripheral neuropathy usually begins peripherally, so that if a person can feel the monofilament on the toes, they do not usually have neuropathy. Isolated areas of apparent insensitivity in other parts of the foot are of much less significance.

Checking foot pulses

The dorsalis pedis and posterior tibial pulses need to be palpated in each foot. They are recorded as either present or absent.

Figure 8.2a
Palpating posterior tibial pulse

Figure 8.2b
Palpating dorsalis pedis pulse

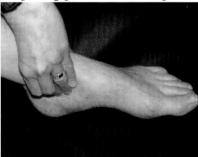

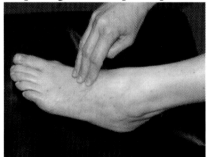

Action to be taken after foot examination

Foot is normal – low current risk of ulceration

Reinforce general foot care education and advice. Give written support information as per Table 8.1. Repeat examination annually.

Table 8.1 General foot care and advice[1]

Self-care and self-monitoring
   • daily examination of the feet for problems (colour change, swelling, breaks in the skin, pain or numbness)
   • footwear (the importance of well-fitting shoes and hosiery)
   • hygiene (daily washing and careful drying)
   • nail care
   • dangers associated with practices such as skin removal (including corn removal)
   • methods to help self examination/monitoring (e.g. the use of mirrors if mobility is limited)

When to seek advice from a health care professional
   • if any colour change, swelling, breaks in the skin, pain or numbness is found
   • if self-care and self-monitoring is not possible or difficult (e.g. because of reduced mobility)

Possible consequences of neglecting the feet
   • foot problems can often be prevented by good diabetes overall management as well as specific foot care
   • prompt detection and management of any problems is important, thus the importance of seeking help as soon as the problem is noticed
   • complications of diabetes such as neuropathy and ischaemia can lead to foot problems such as ulcers, infections, and in extreme cases gangrene and amputation

Foot is abnormal – at-risk (insensitive to monofilament or absent pulses with or without bony abnormality and callus)
   Refer to community diabetes foot care protection team who will:
      • arrange frequent review (1–6 monthly)
      • at each review inspect feet, review need for vascular assessment
      • at each review, evaluate provision of and provide

appropriate intensified foot care education, specialist footwear and insoles, skin and nail care.[1]

People who have at-risk feet should address all the points of education for those with normal feet but in addition need to address the following:

Box 8.1   Education points for those with at-risk feet

- If neuropathy is present, the resulting numbness means that problems may not be noticed, so extra care and vigilance is needed and additional precautions to keep feet protected are needed.
- Do not walk barefoot.
- Seek help to deal with corns and calluses.
- Be aware of the dangers associated with over-the-counter preparations for foot problems (e.g. the danger of corn cures).
- Be aware of potential burning of numb feet, checking bath temperatures, avoiding hot water bottles, electric blankets, foot spas, and sitting too close to fires.
- Moisturise areas of dry skin.
- Regularly check footwear for areas that will cause friction or trauma.
- Seek help from a health care professional if footwear causes difficulties or problems.
- Wear specialist footwear that has been prescribed or supplied.
- Additional advice about foot care on holiday: do not wear new shoes, plan adequate rest periods to avoid additional stress on feet, if flying walk up and down aisles, use sun block on feet – especially on dry skin, take a first aid kit and cover any sore places with sterile dressing, seek help if problems develop, be aware of holiday insurance issues (ensure diabetes cover).

Actions to be taken if foot ulcer or foot infection is found

NICE guidelines[1] recommend that people should be referred to a specialist multidisciplinary diabetes high-risk footcare team within 24 hrs if any of the following occur:

- new ulceration (wound)
- new swelling
- discolouration (redder, bluer, paler, blacker over part or all of foot).

Recommendation level D – evidence from expert committee reports or opinions and/or clinical experience of respected authorities (see Table 2.1, chapter two).

That team as a minimum would be expected to:

- investigate and treat vascular insufficiency
- initiate and supervise wound management – using dressings and debridement as indicated, using systemic antibiotics for cellulitis or bone infection as indicated
- ensure an effective means of distributing foot pressures, including specialist footwear, orthotics and casts
- try to achieve optimal glucose levels and control of risk factors for cardiovascular disease.

Most hospitals now have such foot care teams. They are often co-ordinated by a podiatrist with a special interest in diabetes. It is vital that local GPs and all health care professionals looking after people with diabetes know how to access this team in the emergency situation of discovering a new foot ulcer.

Case history

Ms HY is 38 years old and has had Type 1 diabetes for 24 years. She has had laser treatment for diabetic retinopathy and has lost protective pain sensation in both feet. Her foot pulses were normal. She was methodical about checking her feet and her footwear every day.

She and her partner went abroad for a summer holiday to Turkey. They all wore open sandals as the weather was hot. One afternoon after walking back to the hotel she noticed blood on her sandal. This seemed to arise from an area of blistering and ulceration which contained a small sharp stone and sand.

As they were travelling back home next day she cleaned and dressed the area, and presented to her GP the day after arrival back in the UK. The GP referred her to the multidisciplinary foot care team at the local hospital by contacting the podiatrist in the team and she was seen later that day. The ulcer was treated with debridement, oral broad spectrum antibiotics, and off-loading using special footwear. The ulcer healed in ten weeks.

Ms HY thought that the stone must have got into her sandal as she walked along the water's edge. She said that in future she would always wear trainers on the beach.

Actions for primary care
1. **Ensure that feet are examined at least annually for foot pulses and the presence of neuropathy by using a 10g nylon monofilament.**
   Practice nurses with the special skills and training are well placed to do these examinations, which only take around 90 seconds once shoes and hosiery have been taken off.
2. **Ensure that appropriate education and referral takes place.**
   If foot is not found to be at-risk, practice nurses should give general foot care information, and arrange a re-examination in a year.

   If foot is found to be at-risk, referral is needed to the local community podiatrist for a foot protection programme.

   If foot is ulcerated, or if a person presents with signs of ulceration and/or infection at any other time in the year, an emergency referral needs to be made to the local multidisciplinary foot team for the person to be seen within 24hrs.

Summary points
- People with diabetes are at greatly increased risk of amputation, due to the risk factors of neuropathy and ischaemia.
- Screening for risk factors, extra education and review for those with at-risk feet and prompt referral to a multidisciplinary foot team for those presenting with new ulceration have all been shown to reduce amputation rates.
- Palpating foot pulses and using a 10g nylon monofilament to detect neuropathy are effective screening tests that are quick and easy to use.
- New NICE evidence-based guidelines published in January 2004[1] provide a wealth of evidence to support effective screening and referral in primary care.

References
1. NICE. *CG10 Type 2 diabetes footcare: NICE guideline.* London: NICE, Jan 2004 www.nice.org.uk/pdf/CG010NICEguideline.pdf (accessed 29 Sept 2004)
2. Morris AD, McAlpine R, Steinke D *et al.* Diabetes and lower limb amputations in the community. A retrospective cohort study. DARTS/MEMO Collaboration. *Diabetes Care* 1998; **21**: 738–41
3. Gadsby R , McInnes A. The at-risk foot: the role of the primary care team in achieving St Vincent Targets for reducing amputation. *Diabet Med* 1998; **15(S3)**: S61–64
4. Kumar S, Fernando DJS, Veves A *et al.* Semmes-Weinstein monofilaments: a simple, effective and inexpensive screening device for identifying diabetic patients at risk of foot ulceration. *Diabetes Res Clin Pract* 1991; **13**: 63–8

9 BLOOD PRESSURE CONTROL

Diabetes quality indicator 11 (DM11)
The percentage of patients with diabetes who have a record of the blood pressure in the last 15 months:
Minimum threshold = 25%, maximum threshold to learn full 17 available points = 55%

Diabetes quality indicator 11 (DM12)
The percentage of patients with diabetes in whom the blood pressure is 145/85 or less:
Minimum threshold = 25%, maximum threshold to gain the full 17 available points = 55%

Background

The 17 quality points for hypertension management in diabetes are the largest number available for any one quality indicator. This highlights the importance attached to good blood pressure control in reducing adverse outcomes in diabetes.

Hypertension is positively related to risk of death from cardiovascular disease, with a progressive increase in risk with rising systolic pressures. Reducing blood pressure reduces adverse cardiovascular outcomes. There is a good evidence base for this in people with diabetes.[1]

Evidence base from trials for tight control of blood pressure

The United Kingdom Prospective Diabetes Study (UKPDS) began as a study of glycaemic control in people newly diagnosed with Type 2 diabetes. It then had a blood pressure control study embedded into it.

In the blood pressure study 1148 people with hypertension and Type 2 diabetes were randomised to a tight control arm or a less tight control arm. The final mean difference between the two groups was 10/5 mmHg (144/82 in the tight control group as against 154/87 in the other group). Over nine years those in the tight control group had significant reductions in morbidity and mortality, with:

- 32% reduction in diabetes related death
- 44% reduction in fatal and non fatal stroke
- 56% reduction in congestive cardiac failure
- 37% reduction in developing microvascular complications.

The tightly controlled group were treated with the beta blocker atenolol or the ACE inhibitor captopril, but the study was not sufficiently powered to say which agent was superior.[1] The Hypertension Optimal Treatment Trial (HOT) randomised 18,790 patients with hypertension into three groups – aiming to achieve diastolic pressures of below 90, below 85, and below 80 in each group. The trial contained about 1500 people with Type 2 diabetes. There were significant reductions in cardiovascular morbidity and mortality in the tightest controlled group with a relative risk reduction of 50%.[2]

Recommendations from guidelines on blood pressure targets

The Scottish SIGN evidenced-based guideline 55 on the management of diabetes

This guideline suggests a target level of 140/80 (recommendation level A; see Table 2.1, chapter two).[3]

The 2004 British Hypertension Society guidelines

These recommend a treatment threshold of 140/90 with a target of 140/80 in Type 2 diabetes (recommendation level A – based on category 1 evidence; see Table 2.1, chapter two).[4]

The NICE guideline Management of Type 2 diabetes

On the management of blood pressure and blood lipids NICE recommends a target for treatment of 140/80 or below (recommendation level B – based on category 2 evidence; see Table 2.1, chapter two).[5]

Measuring blood pressure

Box 9.1   Key components of good blood pressure measurement

- subject sitting at rest for 5 mins in quiet surroundings
- arm supported at heart level
- use of appropriately sized cuff
- appropriately calibrated device
- take two separate readings
- record these (and average) to nearest 2 mmHg

In the UKPDS and many other hypertension outcome studies blood pressure was measured with a mercury sphygmomanometer. The use of mercury in medical devices is being phased out due to concerns about its safety by the European Union (EU). Semi-automatic electronic sphygmomanometers are replacing the traditional mercury device in many clinics. It is vital to use one that has been validated by the British Hypertension Society (BHS).[6] Some clinics have stocks of these devices to lend to patients for home blood pressure monitoring. As they become cheaper some patients are buying their own. It is also possible that devices for continuous ambulatory blood pressure monitoring will come in to more widespread use in the next few years.

Home blood pressure monitoring with its multiple measurements over time may be found to give better prognostic information than isolated clinic readings.[7] However, we need to remember that the thresholds and targets upon which blood pressure management is based in the quality payment scheme are derived from research studies where the clinic measurements were usually made with mercury devices.

Treating raised blood pressure

Trial evidence suggests that achieving blood pressure reductions to target levels is more important than which individual drug therapy is used. In the UKPDS blood pressure study,[1] after nine years of follow up 29%

Figure 9.1   Measuring blood pressure

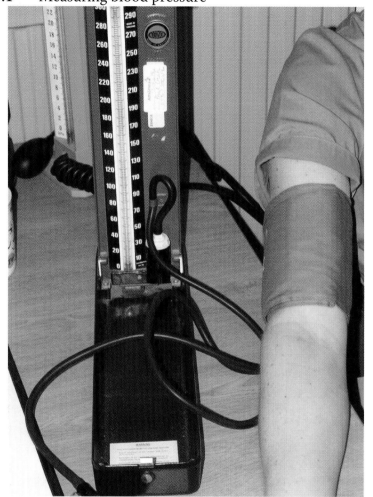

of people in the tight control group needed three or more therapies to meet target blood pressure. Indeed, in practice many people with Type 2 diabetes will not have their blood pressure controlled to target on one therapy alone. This means that the controversies over which is the best agent to use as initial monotherapy are rather superfluous. It is known that the concordance with therapy decreases with increasing numbers of tablets and increasing dose frequency.[8] It is likely, therefore, that combination therapy will be needed to reduce numbers of tablets that people need to take. Low dose diuretics augment the antihypertensive effects of other major classes and so diuretic–beta blocker or diuretic–ACE inhibitor combinations may help.

Box 9.2 NICE recommendations on choice of agent to reduce blood pressure[5]

- Use ACE inhibitors, angiotensin 2 receptor blockers (ARB2), beta blockers or thiazide diuretics as first line treatments in people who do not have microalbuminuria (evidence level A).
- Long-acting dihydropyridine and non-dihydropyridine calcium channel blockers have an important role in treating blood pressure, but on current evidence should be prescribed as second line treatment or as part of combination therapy (evidence level B).
- Do not prescribe short-acting calcium channel blockers (evidence level D).
- Anticipate that combination therapy with any or all of these drug classes will be required to meet treatment targets in the majority of people (evidence level C).
- Assess the response to treatment frequently (every 3–6 months when stabilised, more frequently when titrating treatment).

Pragmatic therapy action plan based on the above

Step one
ACE inhibitor (or if not tolerated ARB2) or thiazide

Step two
Add in the agent not used in step one

Step three
Add beta blocker

Step four
Add long-acting dihydropyridone or non-dihydropyridine calcium channel blocker

Step five
Add alpha blocker

Blood pressure treatment when there is microalbuminuria or proteinuria

Microalbuminuria is the leakage of protein from the kidney of 30 to 300mg in 24 hours. Proteinuria is the leakage of more than 300mg in 24 hours. In Type 2 diabetes most people with microalbuminuria will have raised blood pressure. The presence of microalbuminuria doubles the risk of cardiovascular disease. It has been argued that people with microalbuminuria should be targeted for intensive risk reduction and have a lower target blood pressure. The NICE guideline[5] suggests a target of 135/75 (evidence level B) and states that ACE inhibitors should be the class of first choice to treat people with microalbuminuria or proteinuria (evidence level A).

Trial evidence for ARB2s

Several recent studies have looked at the role of ARB2 therapy in people with Type 2 diabetes and microalbuminuria or proteinuria. In the IRMA-2 study[8] irbesartan decreased progression to overt nephropathy in people with microalbuminuria by 70% compared with placebo, despite a difference of only 3 mmHg in systolic blood pressure in the treatment compared with placebo group. The IDNT study[9] was conducted in people with nephropathy with proteinuria of greater than 900mg in 24 hours. Irbesartan was found to be superior to both placebo and amlodipine (in combination with other antihypertensive agents) in preventing a doubling of serum creatinine. The RENAAL study[10] looked at losartan versus placebo in combination with other conventional antihypertensive agents in those with Type 2 diabetes and proteinuria of greater than 500mg in 24 hours. Losartan treatment was associated with a 16% reduction in the primary endpoint, which was a composite of doubling of creatinine progression to end-stage renal failure (ESRD) and death. These trials give the ARB2 agents irbesartan and losartan a specific evidence base in people with Type 2 diabetes and nephropathy.

Combining ACE and ARB2 therapy

Further trials of the benefits and safety of such combinations are awaited but a preliminary study in people with Type 2 diabetes, hypertension and microalbuminuria support this use.[11]

Using exception reporting

As with glycaemia targets there are some people for whom it would be inappropriate to try to attain the target BP of 145/85, and some in whom it is impossible. The Read code 8BL0.00 can be used for exception reporting. It is a code for maximum tolerated doses of antihypertensive agents. People for whom it may be necessary to use this code include the terminally ill, the frail elderly who are at extra risk of falling and fracturing bones, and people who get postural hypotension symptoms when blood pressure levels are reduced towards the target.

Case history

Ms GH, a 53-year-old woman who has had Type 2 diabetes for two years. She is controlled on diet and exercise. She has had hypertension for five years and her diabetes was diagnosed through the screening of people with hypertension. She has been on bendrofluazide 2.5mg daily for five years. Her BP being 160/90, she was started on an ACE inhibitor ramipril, beginning with 2.5mg and titrating up to 10mg daily. Her urea and electrolytes were monitored and remained within the normal range.

On 10mg ramipril and 2.5 bendrofluazide her BP settled to 140/80. She had no microalbuminuria.

Actions for primary care
1. Measure blood pressure accurately at each diabetes consultation. Record the level using the appropriate Read code.
2. Practice nurses with special training and skills in diabetes management may be the best people to measure blood pressure.
3. If blood pressure hasn't reached target level of 145/85 and further lowering is appropriate titrate up dose of current agent, or move to next treatment step and add new agent.
4. Plan to review in a few weeks to monitor the effect of the therapy change, and repeat step 2 (see page 93).

Summary points
- Hypertension and diabetes frequently co-exist.
- Reducing blood pressure improves adverse outcomes.
- Blood pressure lowering is more important than the specific agent used.
- A significant number of people will require two or more agents to reach the target of 145/85.
- Regular measurement of blood pressure with therapy dose adjustment will enable the quality points targets for blood pressure to be achieved.

References
1. UKPDS Group. Tight blood pressure control and risk of macrovascular and microvascular complications in Type 2 diabetes (UKPDS 38). *BMJ* 1998; **317**: 703–13
2. Hansson L, Zanchetti A, Carruthers SG *et al.* Effects of intensive blood pressure lowering and low dose aspirin therapy in patients with hypertension. Principal results of the Hypertension Optimal Treatment (HOT) randomised trial. *Lancet* 1998; **351**: 1755–62
3. Scottish Intercollegiate Guidelines Network. *Management of Diabetes: SIGN guideline 55.* Edinburgh: SIGN, Nov 2001 www.sign.ac.uk/guidelines/fulltext/55/index.html (accessed 30 Sept 2004)
4. Ramsey LE, Williams B, Johnston GD *et al.* British Hypertension Society guidelines for hypertension management (BHS- IV): Summary. *BMJ* 2004; **328**: 634–40
5. NICE. *Management of Type 2 Diabetes – management of blood*

pressure and blood lipids (Guideline H) London: NICE, 2002. www.nice.org.uk/page.aspx?o=38551 (accessed 30 Sept 2004)

6. British Hypertension Society. Revised BHS protocol for the evaluation of measuring devices. *J Hypertens* 1993; **11:** S43–62

7. Petrie J. Blood pressure measurement in diabetes: theory and practice. *British Journal of Diabetes and Vascular Disease* 2003; **3:** 258–61

8. Parving HH, Lehnert H Brochner-Mortensen J *et al.* The effect of irbesartan on the development of diabetic nephropathy in patients with type 2 diabetes. *New Engl J Med* 2001; **345:** 870–8

9. Lewis EJ, Hunsicker LG, Clarke WR *et al.* The angiotensin receptor antagonist irbesartan in patients with nephropathy due to type 2 diabetes. New Engl J Med 2001 **345:** 851–60

10. Brenner BM, Cooper ME, de Zeeuw D *et al.* Effects of Losartan on renal and cardiovascular outcomes in patients with type 2 diabetes and nephropathy. *New Engl J Med* 2001; **345:** 861–9

11. Morgensen CE, Neldham S Tikkanen I *et al.* Randomised controlled trial of dual blockade of rennin-angiotensin system in patients with hypertension, microalbuminuria, and non insulin dependant diabetes: the candasartan and lisinopril microalbuminuria (CALM) study. *BMJ* 2000; **321:** 868–73

Diabetes quality indicator 13 (DM 13)
The percentage of patients with diabetes who have a record of microalbuminuria testing in the previous 15 months (exception reporting for patients with proteinuria):
Minimum threshold = 25%, maximum threshold to earn maximum 3 points = 90%

Diabetes quality indicator 14 (DM 14)
The percentage of patients with diabetes who have a record of serum creatinine testing in the previous 15 months:
Minimum threshold = 25%, maximum threshold to earn maximum 3 points = 90%

Diabetes quality indicator (DM 15)
The percentage of patients with diabetes with proteinuria or microalbuminuria who are treated with Angiotensin Converting Enzyme (ACE) inhibitors (or Angiotensin 2 Receptor Blockers (ARB2):
Minimum threshold = 25%, maximum threshold to earn maximum 3 points = 70%

Definitions
Proteinuria is defined as the leakage into the urine of greater than 300mg protein in 24 hours. This amount of protein leakage will mean that the urine tests positive on a proteinuria urine testing stick. It is sometimes labelled as dip-stick positive proteinuria. Albustix and Medi-Test Protein 2 are two protein-testing strips that are available in the UK. Proteinuria testing is found as part of various branded combination sticks e.g. uristix, multistix etc.
Microalbuminuria is defined as the leakage into the urine of protein in the range 30–300mg in 24 hours and can be detected by the Micral-Test strip. The urine will test negative to normal protein dip-sticks.
Normoalbuminuria is defined as the leakage into the urine of less than 30mg protein in 24 hours.
Diabetic nephropathy is defined as renal disease caused by diabetes mellitus.

The natural history of the development of nephropathy in Type 1 diabetes

Not everyone with Type 1 diabetes will develop nephropathy, but in those that do a progressive natural history has been described. In the first few years of living with diabetes, kidney function is normal and there is variable excretion of only tiny amounts of protein, less than 30mg in 24 hours. Later, often after from eight to ten years of living with diabetes, microalbuminuria may develop. This stage may last for ten years. People at this stage usually have a normal blood pressure.

From approximately 20 years onwards of living with diabetes, frank proteinuria may develop. This continues on with progressive renal impairment, a rising serum creatinine level, hypertension and can lead to the need for renal replacement therapy (dialysis or transplantation) after approximately 25–30 years of living with diabetes. The cumulative incidence of microalbuminuria in patients with Type 1 diabetes for 30 years is around 40%.[1] Around 20% of people with Type 1 diabetes develop proteinuria after 25 years of living with diabetes.[2]

Trial evidence for interventions in Type 1 diabetes

In the Diabetes Control and Complications Trial (DCCT) involving 1400 people with Type 1 diabetes,[3] a reduction in mean HbA1c from 9% in the standard treatment group to 7% in the intensive treatment group was associated with a 39% reduction in the occurrence of microalbuminuria and a 54% reduction in proteinuria over a mean of 6.5 years. After completion of the trial the participants were followed up. Glycaemic control in the two groups rapidly converged to a mean HbA1c of 8%. However, persistent beneficial effects on albumin excretion and a reduced incidence of hypertension have been noted in those who were in the intensively controlled group as compared with those in the standard control group, indicating that intensive glycaemic control even for a limited time has long-term benefits.[4]

ACE inhibitors, when given to people with Type 1 diabetes who are normotensive but who have microalbuminuria, can delay or postpone the progression of nephropathy.[5] Most published studies of ACE therapy showing these benefits have been at the higher end of their therapeutic dose ranges.

Natural history in Type 2 diabetes

In Type 2 diabetes most people with microalbuminuria also have hypertension. The presence of microalbuminuria is a marker for increased cardiovascular risk, and a number of people with microalbuminuria will die of coronary heart disease before they have time to develop end-stage renal disease.

Trial evidence for interventions in Type 2 diabetes

In the United Kingdom Prospective Diabetes Study (UKPDS) study[6] of over 5000 people with newly diagnosed Type 2 diabetes, a reduction in mean HbA1c from 7.9% in the standard treatment group to 7% in the intensive treatment group was associated with an absolute risk reduction of developing microalbuminuria of 11%, proteinuria of 3.5% and a twofold increase in serum creatinine of 2.5%. Good glycaemic control clearly reduces the risk of nephropathy in Type 2 diabetes.

Treatment with an ACE inhibitor is also beneficial. In one study, treatment with the ACE inhibitor ramipril, in people with Type 2 diabetes for a mean of 4.5 years, reduced cardiovascular mortality by 25% in people with normal serum creatinine levels and in those with mild renal insufficiency.[7]

Several studies have also shown the benefit of angiotensin 2 antagonists (AT2s). In one study, 5% of Type 2 patients with microalbuminuria developed diabetic nephropathy when treated with irbesartan, compared to 15% in a control group, over two years. This effect was independent of blood pressure.[8] At the stage of diabetic nephropathy with a reduced glomerular filtration rate,

17% of Type 2 patients treated with irbesartan doubled their serum creatinine level over 2.6 years in contrast to 25% in a control group.[9]

Statements from guidelines

The SIGN guidelines[10] state:

- All patients with diabetes should have their urinary albumin concentration and serum creatinine measured at diagnosis and at regular intervals, usually annually.
- Urinary albumin concentration should be measured using a first morning urine sample and the urinary albumin:creatinine ratio should be measured by a laboratory method or a near-patient test specific for microalbuminuria.
- Patients with microalbuminuria or proteinuria should be commenced on an ACE inhibitor.
- Patients should be referred to a renal clinic if serum creatinine exceeds 150 mmol/l.

The NICE guidelines[11] state:

For people with higher-risk urine albumin excretion (i.e. microalbuminuria or proteinuria):

- begin therapy with an appropriate ACE inhibitor
- maintain BP below 135/75
- refer for specialist/nephrology opinion if serum creatinine level exceeds 150.

Detecting microalbuminuria

Microalbuminuria can occur in healthy people after they have been standing for a while, that is why tests are done after a period of recumbence, usually after sleep. It can occur after exercise or during a febrile illness. Near-patient testing strips are available to be used to detect microalbuminuria. They are dipped into the urine and undergo a colour change if microalbuminuria is present. It can be detected in a urine sample sent to a laboratory for the detection of the albumin:creatinine ratio (A:C).

A ratio greater than 2.5mg / mmol for men and 3.5 for women indicates microalbuminuria.

If either the stick test or the A:C ratio is normal the patient can be left for a repeat check in one year.

If the stick test or the A:C ratio is abnormal the NICE guideline states that they need to be repeated twice within a month and, if two out of three tests are positive, microalbuminuria is said to be present.

Non-diabetic causes of proteinuria or microalbuminuria

The microvascular complications of diabetes tend to occur together. If microalbuminuria or proteinuria is detected and the person does not have retinopathy non-diabetic causes of the abnormal protein excretion need to be investigated. Such investigations might need to include renal ultrasound and an intravenous pyelogram (IVP).

Actions for primary care

1. Measure serum creatinine as part of the diabetes annual review blood tests.
2. Dipstick the urine for protein annually.
3. In those who are Albustix negative, check for microalbuminuria using a near-patient test or by sending a urine sample to the laboratory for an A:C ratio.
4. If the A:C ratio is also negative repeat the process annually.
5. If either test is positive, repeat it twice. Two out of three positives confirms that microalbuminuria has been detected.
6. Ensure that those who have proteinuria or microalbuminuria are on full dose ACE inhibitor therapy. If ACE is not tolerated use AT2.
7. Maintain blood pressure below 135/75.
8. Ensure optimal glycaemic control.

Case history

> Mr TR is 32 and has had Type 1 diabetes for 17 years. His HbA1c is 6.9% and his blood pressure is 136/80 in the absence of antihypertensive treatment.
>
> As part of his annual diabetes review two years ago he tested positive for microalbuminuria. As a result of this he was started on the ACE inhibitor lisinopril, initially at 2.5mg daily. The dose was titrated up to 20mg with regular monitoring of blood pressure and urea, electrolytes and creatinine. His blood pressure has remained virtually unchanged (in the range 132–138/76–80) and there has been no progression of the microalbuminuria. Serum creatinine has remained stable at 86.

Summary points

- The natural history of nephropathy progressing through microalbuminuria to frank proteinuria and end-stage renal failure in Type 1 diabetes has been well-described.
- ACE inhibitor treatment can delay this progression in people with Type 1 diabetes and microalbuminuria who do not usually have hypertension, as can intensive glycaemic control (HbA1c 7% or below).
- ACE inhibitor therapy and treatment with ARB2s can delay progression of nephropathy in Type 2 diabetes, as can intensive glycaemic control (HbA1c 7% or below).

References

1. Parving HH, Hommel E, Mathiesen E *et al.* Prevalence of microalbuminuria, arterial hypertension, retinopathy and neuropathy in patients with insulin dependant diabetes mellitus. *BMJ* 1988; **296:** 156–60
2. Microvascular and acute complications in IDDM patients; the EURODIAB IDDM Complications Study. *Diabetologia* 1994; **37:** 278–85
3. The effect of intensive treatment of diabetes on the development and progression of long-term complications in insulin-dependent diabetes mellitus. The Diabetes Control and Complications Research Group (DCCT). *N Engl J Med* 1993; **329:** 977–86
4. Writing Team for the Diabetes Control and Complications Trial/Epidemiology of Diabetes Interventions and Complications Research Group. Sustained effect of intensive treatment of type 1 diabetes mellitus on

development and progression of diabetic nephropathy: the Epidemiology of Diabetes Interventions and Complications (EDIC) study. *JAMA* 2003; **290:** 2159–67

5. Mathiesen E, Hommel E, Giesel J *et al.* Efficacy of Captopril in postponing nephropathy in normotensive insulin dependant diabetic patients with microalbuminuria. *BMJ* 1991; **303:** 81–7

6. UK Prospective Diabetes Study group. Intensive blood glucose control with sulphonylureas or insulin compared with conventional treatment and risk of complications in patients with Type 2 diabetes (UKPDS 33). *Lancet* 1998; **352:** 837–53

7. Heart Outcomes Prevention Evaluation Study Investigators. Effects of ramipril on cardiovascular and microvascular outcomes in people with diabetes melitus; results of the HOPE study and MICRO-HOPE substudy. *Lancet* 2000; **355:** 253–9

8. Parving HH, Lehnert H, Brocher-Mortensen J *et al.* The effect of irbesartan on the development of diabetic nephropathy in patients with type 2 diabetes. *N Engl J Med* 2001; **345:** 870–8

9. Lewis EJ, Hunsicker LG, Clarke WR *et al.* Renoprotective effect of the angiotensin-receptor antagonist irbesartan in patients with nephropathy due to type 2 diabetes. *N Engl J Med* 2001; **345:** 851–60

10. Scottish Intercollegiate Guidelines Network. *Management of Diabetes* Edinburgh: SIGN, Nov 2001 (SIGN guideline 55) www.sign.ac.uk/guidelines/fulltext/55/index.html (accessed 30 Sept 2004)

11. NICE. *Management of Type 2 diabetes. Renal disease – prevention and early management. Inherited guideline F.* London: NICE, 2002 www.nice.org.uk/page.aspx?o=27964 (accessed 30 Sept 2004)

Diabetes quality indicator (DM 16)

The percentage of patients with diabetes who have a record of total cholesterol in the previous 15 months:

Minimum threshold = 25%, maximum threshold to earn full available 3 points = 90%

Diabetes quality indicator (DM 17)

The percentage of patients with diabetes whose last measured total cholesterol within previous 15 months is 5 mmol/l or less:

Minimum threshold = 25%, maximum threshold to earn full available 3 points = 60%

Background

Cardiovascular disease risk is increased from two- to fourfold in Type 2 diabetes. Seventy-five per cent of people with Type 2 diabetes will die of cardiovascular disease and life expectancy is reduced by approximately ten years by Type 2 diabetes.[1] There is good evidence that therapy with a statin will reduce total serum cholesterol levels and will also reduce adverse cardiovascular events. There has been much debate as to whether it is important to measure high density (HDL) and low density (LDL) cholesterol components and triglyceride levels, which have to be measured in a fasting blood sample. The quality standards of the new contract simplify matters by only being concerned with total cholesterol measurements that can be performed on a random (non-fasting) blood sample.

A distinction can also be made between primary and secondary coronary heart disease (CHD) prevention. With primary prevention there are no signs or symptoms of pre-existing CHD. Secondary prevention is required for people who have already had a myocardial infarction, stroke, peripheral vascular disease or angina.

The quality standards again simplify matters by not making these distinctions. They also do not distinguish between Type 2 diabetes where there is a lot of evidence, and Type 1 diabetes where there is less.

Some guidelines have suggested that treatment with a statin be related to the overall CHD risk score as calculated from a risk calculator, e.g. the CHD risk calculator of the Joint British Societies,[2] rather than just to a total cholesterol level. This risk calculator is based on data from the Framingham Study, whose population was largely Caucasian in ethnic background and contained few people with diabetes. Many GP clinical computer systems have it pre-installed, and the charts are found in the back of the British National Formulary (BNF). It tends therefore to under-estimate CHD risk in people with Type 2 diabetes. It is also not applicable to people with Type 1 diabetes, to those from Indo-Asian ethnic backgrounds and to people with Type 2 diabetes and microalbuminuria (who are at significantly increased risk). Again, the quality standards simplify matters by dealing only with cholesterol measurements and targeting a level of 5 mmol/l or below for all people with diabetes.

Evidence from trials for cholesterol lowering in diabetes

Several clinical trials have demonstrated the efficacy of statins for cholesterol lowering and CHD risk reduction in general populations. Although the proportions of subjects diagnosed with diabetes included in the final analyses from these studies were relatively low (varying from 1% to 15%), sub-group analyses show that intensive cholesterol lowering can reduce the incidence of cardiovascular events in these patients.

The Prospective Pravastatin Pooling (PPP) project[3] pooled data from the Current And Recurrent Events (CARE) trial,[4] the West Of Scotland Coronary Prevention Study (WOSCOPS)[5] and the Long-Term Intervention with Pravastatin in Ischaemic Disease (LIPID)

Study[6] and demonstrated that pravastatin therapy reduced the incidence of coronary events in patients with and without diabetes. The Heart Protection Study (HPS)[7] examined data from 5963 patients with diabetes (29% of all patients studied) and demonstrated that the incidence of major vascular events in these patients was reduced by 20% with simvastatin 40mg compared with placebo; this reduction was similar to that observed for the entire study population. This study enrolled people with total cholesterol levels above 3.5 mmol/l. The results of the HPS suggest that it is statin treatment rather than reduction of cholesterol to any specific arbitrary figure that produces the benefit.

In the CARDS study 2838 people with Type 2 diabetes, aged from 40 to 75 years and from 132 centres around the UK, were randomised to placebo or atorvastatin 10mg daily. Study entrants had no history of CHD, an LDL cholesterol of 4.14 mmol or lower, and at least one of the following conditions: retinopathy, albuminuria, current smoking, or hypertension. The trial was stopped two years earlier than expected because the pre-specified early stopping rule for efficacy had been met. The median duration of follow up was 3.9 years.

In the placebo group, 127 people had one major CHD event (acute coronary disease event, coronary revascularisation or stroke), in contrast to 83 people in the atorvastatin group. The risk reduction with atorvastatin for a CHD event was 37%. Atorvastatin reduced the death rate by 27%. No excess of adverse events was noted in the atorvastatin group.

The authors conclude that atorvastatin is safe and efficacious in reducing the risk of first CHD events in people with Type 2 diabetes without a high LDL cholesterol. They also conclude that no justification is available for having a particular threshold level of LDL cholesterol as the sole arbiter by which patients with Type 2 diabetes should receive statins. The debate about whether all people with Type 2 diabetes warrant statin treatment should now focus on whether any patients are at a sufficiently low risk for the treatment to be withheld.

All the statin studies published so far suggest that people with diabetes gain at least as much benefit from statin therapy as people without diabetes. However, because the relative risk of CHD is two- to fourfold higher, the absolute benefit of statin therapy is likely to be greater.

What guidelines recommend

The SIGN[8] guidelines state:

If total cholesterol is greater than 5 mmol/l, statin therapy to reduce total cholesterol should be initiated and titrated as necessary to reduce total cholesterol to below 5.

The NICE guidelines on management of blood pressure and blood lipids[9]

These guidelines have much more complicated recommendations for the pharmacological management of adverse blood lipid profiles in people with Type 2 diabetes, based on levels of total cholesterol or LDL cholesterol, triglycerides, whether it is primary or secondary prevention and ten-year risk of a coronary event taken from a risk calculator. These were published before the HPS study was and therefore do not reflect information from that important trial.

Which statin to use to lower cholesterol

The trial evidence base for reducing adverse CHD outcomes in people with diabetes through cholesterol lowering by prescribing a statin comes largely from studies that used pravastatin at 40mg daily or simvastatin at 40mg daily or atorvastatin 10mg daily.

What to add to statin if the target of 5 mmol/l is not achieved

It is possible to add a fibrate to the statin to lower cholesterol further. Fibrates are also useful agents if triglyceride levels are significantly elevated. The efficacy and tolerability of statin-fibrate combinations have been examined in people with a high risk of CHD, but there is only limited data available from studies in people with diabetes.[10] Safety concerns surrounding the tolerability of particular statin–fibrate combinations have led many to re-evaluate prescribing these combinations. Reports of deaths attributable to drug-related rhabdomylosis with cerivastatin administered in high doses or in combination with the fibrate gemfibrozil, led to the recent withdrawl of cerivastatin from the market.[10] The risk of adverse events appears to be much more common with cerivastatin than other statins. However, it is recommended that statin–fibrate combination therapy should be used with caution and patients receiving such combination therapy require close monitoring for signs of muscle and liver toxicity.[10]

The drug ezetimibe, a cholesterol absorption inhibitor, has been recently released. When added to a statin, it can give further reductions in total cholesterol levels. As it is very new its precise role in cholesterol management in diabetes remains to be determined.

Sustained-release nicotinamide has also been shown to lower cholesterol. It can be used in combination with a statin.

Actions for primary care
1. Measure total cholesterol as part of the annual review blood tests.
2. Encourage people with diabetes to eat a low fat diet as part of healthy eating advice.
3. Give statin therapy to people with diabetes who have a raised cholesterol and aim to lower their total cholesterol to below 5 mmol/l.
4. If full dose statin therapy does not reduce the total cholesterol to below 5 mmol/l consider adding a fibrate, or consider the agent ezetimibe. Closely monitor people on statin–fibrate combinations for signs of toxicity.

Summary points

- People with diabetes are at increased risk of CHD.
- Although data from studies in people with diabetes is limited, it appears that statin therapy is effective in lowering total cholesterol and protecting against adverse CHD outcomes in both primary and secondary prevention.
- Measuring total cholesterol as part of the annual review blood tests and treating people with raised cholesterol levels with a statin should enable the full quality points to be achieved.

References

1. Donnelly R, Emsie-Smith AM, Gardner IS, Morris AD. ABC of arterial and vascular disease. Vascular complications of diabetes. *BMJ* 2000; **320**: 1062–6
2. Joint British Societies Coronary Risk Prediction Charts. *Heart* 1998; **80**: S1–S29
3. Sacks FM, Tonkin AM, Shepherd J *et al*. Effect of pravastatin on coronary disease events in subgroups defined by coronary risk factors: the Prospective Pravastatin Pooling Project Investigators Group. *Circulation* 2000; **102**: 1893–900
4. Sacks FM, Pfeffer MA, Moye LA *et al*. The effect of pravastatin on coronary events after myocardial infarction in patients with average cholesterol levels. Cholesterol and Recurrent Events Trial Investigators. *N Engl J Med* 1996; **335**: 1001–9
5. Shepherd J, Cobbe SM, Ford I *et al*. Prevention of coronary heart disease with pravastatin in men with hypercholesterolemia. West of Scotland Coronary Prevention Study Group. *N Engl J Med* 1995; **333**: 1301–7
6. The Long-Term Intervention with Pravastatin in Ischaemic Disease (LIPID) Study Group. Prevention of cardiovascular events and death with pravastatin in patients with coronary heart disease and a broad range of initial cholesterol levels. *N Engl J Med* 1998; **339**: 1349–57
7. Heart Protection Study Group. MRC/BHF Heart Protection Study of cholesterol lowering with simvastatin in 20,536 high-risk individuals: a randomised placebo-controlled trial. *Lancet* 2002; **360**: 7–22
8. Scottish Intercollegiate Guidelines Network. *Management of Diabetes*. Edinburgh: SIGN, Nov 2001 (SIGN guideline 55) www.sign.ac.uk/guidelines/fulltext/55/index.html (accessed 30 Sept 2004)
9. NICE. *Management of Type 2 Diabetes – management of blood pressure and blood lipids (Guideline H)* London: NICE, 2002. www.nice.org.uk/page.aspx?o=38551 (accessed 30 Sept 2004)
10. Gadsby R Diabetic dyslipidaemia – the case for using statins. *British Journal of Diabetes and Vascular Disease* 2003; **3**: 402–7

Influenza Immunisation

Diabetes quality indicator 18 (DM 18)
The percentage of patients with diabetes who have had an influenza immunisation in the preceding 1 September to 31 March:
Minimum threshold = 25%, maximum threshold to achieve the full 3 points = 85%

Background

Outbreaks of influenza have been recognised since ancient times and are responsible for devastating global morbidity and mortality. The 1989–90 epidemic was responsible for 29,000 deaths in the UK.[1] Chronic illness, including diabetes are said to be risk factors for influenza morbidity and mortality. Annual influenza vaccination is recommended in the UK for everyone with diabetes.

Evidence for influenza immunisation in people with diabetes

Excess deaths during an influenza epidemic have been attributed mostly to respiratory infections and cardiovascular causes.[2] They are mainly in the age group of over 60 years. Most studies have confirmed that high-risk subjects with chronic diseases (cardiovascular or respiratory diseases, renal failure, and diabetes mellitus) considered together as one group, have a three to four times excess mortality from influenza than people without chronic diseases.[2] Most studies have not included sufficient numbers of people with diabetes to allow the contribution of diabetes *per se* to be examined with confidence. During the 1989–90 epidemic, morbidity from bronchitis was significantly increased in people with chronic illness and specifically in people with diabetes.[3] Rates of admission to hospital of people with diabetic ketoacidosis are increased during an influenza epidemic.[4]

A large body of evidence suggests that influenza

immunisation, when the vaccine composition match-
es that of the infecting agent, significantly reduces the
mortality associated with influenza. This is particularly
true in older subjects.[5] There are no clinical studies specifically examining the clinical effectiveness of influenza
immunisation in people with diabetes, but there are no
reasons to suggest that the vaccine is less effective in
this group. In the general population influenza immunisation is cost effective,[5] especially in older people.[6]
Again, there are no cost-effectiveness studies address-
ing this issue directly in people with diabetes, but there
are likewise no reasons to suppose that it would not be
cost effective in this group.

Statements from guidelines

There are no specific statements about influenza vaccination in the Type 2 NICE guideline series or in the
SIGN guidelines. The American Diabetes Association
(ADA) recommends that influenza immunisation be
recommended for people with diabetes aged over six
months, beginning each September. It states that this
view is based largely on observational studies with a
high potential for bias, but that expert opinion supports
the view that influenza immunisation is a low-risk, low-
cost intervention that may have a moderate to substantial impact on the care of people with diabetes.[7]

Side effects of influenza immunisation

The influenza vaccine contains only non-infectious
viruses and cannot cause influenza or other respiratory disease. The side effect most usually reported is
mild soreness at the vaccination site. In individuals
with chicken egg allergy immediate allergic reactions
have been reported, so influenza immunisation should
be avoided in these people. It is also suggested that it
should not be given to anyone known to have developed
Guillain-Barré syndrome within six weeks of a previous
influenza immunisation.[7]

Practical steps to be taken

Opportunistic

People attending diabetes clinics in the practice from September through to December can be opportunistically offered immunisation at that visit. Unfortunately this will only cover a small proportion of those at risk.

By invitation

Many practices will have developed a system of call and recall to offer influenza immunisation to their at-risk patients. This usually takes the form of a letter sent to individuals in September inviting them to attend for an influenza immunisation at a specific time. Such immunisations may be done by practice nurses and other health care professionals in special clinics or in normal practice nurse surgery times. Special arrangements are usually made to immunise those who are housebound or who live in residential or nursing homes. This may involve the community nursing team or immunisation as part of a GP home visit.

In my experience, people over 65 (who are likely to make up over 50% of the practice diabetes population) are getting the message that influenza immunisation is important. It is younger people, especially those with Type 1 diabetes in their twenties and thirties, who often do not see the need. Many of these will be attending hospital clinics for their diabetes follow up. We will need the help and assistance of our colleagues in secondary care to remind these people of the value of influenza immunisation.

Exclusion reporting

Some people choose not to have the influenza immunisation for various personal reasons, and a few may have egg allergy. They may be excluded from the total population, from whom the 25% minimum threshold and the 85% maximum thresholds are derived by using the appropriate exclusion code: declined influenza vaccine = 8I2S, influenza vaccine contraindicated = 9OX5.

Summary points

- Expert opinion supports the view that influenza immunisation is a low-risk, low-cost, useful intervention for all people with diabetes over six months of age.
- Opportunistic and invitation-based immunisation programmes are needed every autumn to achieve this quality payment.

References

1. Ashley J, Smith T, Dunnel K. Deaths in Great Britain associated with the influenza epidemic of 1989–90. *Population Trends.* London: HMSO 1991; **65:** 16–20

2. Barker WH, Mullooly JP. Impact of epidemic Type A influenza in a defined adult population. *Am J Epidemiol* 1980; **112:** 798–811

3. Connolly AM, Salmon RL, Lervy B *et al.* What are the complications of influenza and can they be prevented? Experience from the 1989 epidemic of H3N2 influenza A in general practice. *BMJ* 1993; **306:** 1452–4

4. Watkins P, Soler NG, Fitzgerald MG Malins JM. Diabetic ketoacidosis during an influenza epidemic. *BMJ* 1970; **4:** 89–91

5. Nichol KL, Margolis KL, Wuorenma J *et al.* The efficacy and cost effectiveness of vaccination against influenza among elderly persons living in the community. *N Engl J Med* 1994; **331:** 778–84.

6. Perez-Tirse J. Gross PA Review of the cost-benefit analysis of influenza vaccine. *Pharmacoeconomics* 1992; **2:** 198–206

7. American Diabetes Association Immunisation and the prevention of Influenza and Pneumococcal Disease in people with Diabetes. *Diabetes Care* 2003; **26:** S126–8

13 PREGNANCY AND GESTATIONAL DIABETES

There are many other aspects of diabetes care that are not covered by quality standards. Some aspects of diabetes care are more difficult to count. That does not make them any less important than the ones that can! It is very important for GPs and the primary care diabetes team to be aware of them and to practice good evidence-based care in these areas too. This chapter deals with the important subject of pregnancy and gestational diabetes.

Diabetes and pregnancy

The *National Service Framework for Diabetes: Standards* has one specific standard for diabetes and pregnancy in Standard 9, which says:

> *The NHS will develop, implement and monitor policies that seek to empower and support women with pre-existing diabetes and those who develop diabetes during pregnancy to optimise outcomes of their pregnancy.*

What is the evidence showing that good care reduces adverse outcomes?

There is evidence that the infants of women with diabetes who attend multidisciplinary pre-pregnancy counselling show significantly fewer major congenital malformations compared with infants of non-attending mothers. The attending mothers also have fewer pregnancy complications.[1]

Optimal blood glucose control before and during pregnancy reduces congenital malformations, stillbirth, neonatal hypoglycaemia and respiratory distress syndrome. Blood glucose levels around conception and during the pregnancy should be between 4 and 7 mmol. This is likely to require intensive blood glucose monitoring and intensive insulin therapy.[2] Established diabetic retinal and renal disease can deteriorate during pregnancy. It is important to examine the retinae of a pregnant woman during each trimester. More frequent assessment may be required in those with poor glycaemic control or hypertension.[2]

Gestational diabetes

Gestational diabetes (GDM) is carbohydrate intolerance with onset or first recognition during pregnancy, and includes women with abnormal glucose tolerance that reverts to normal after pregnancy, and those with Type 1 and Type 2 diabetes newly diagnosed in pregnancy. All pregnant women need to have a urine test for glycosuria at each antenatal clinic attendance and need to have an OGTT if GDM is suspected. There is still no consensus on the most appropriate methods for screening, diagnosing and managing asymptomatic GDM.[2]

There are a number of ways of screening for gestational diabetes practised in different units in the UK. One pragmatic approach is to test the urine for glucose at each antenatal visit with the addition of a timed random laboratory plasma glucose measurement at booking, 28 weeks' gestation and whenever glycosuria is detected.[3]

There is a risk of up to 50% of future diabetes in women who develop GDM, and babies of mothers with GDM have an increased risk of perinatal morbidity. There is some evidence for improved perinatal morbidity through screening and early detection of GDM, but there is also an increased caesarean section rate. Despite its limitations, the OGTT has become established as the 'most acceptable' screening test for GDM.[4]

What the guidelines say

The SIGN guidelines

- Pre-pregnancy care provided by a multidisciplinary team is strongly recommended for women with diabetes.

- All women with diabetes should be prescribed pre-pregnancy folate supplementation, continuing up to 12 weeks' gestation.
- Before and during pregnancy, women with diabetes should aim to have blood glucose between 4 and 7 mmol/l.

Actions for primary care

1. **Pre-pregnancy counselling**

    Such counselling needs to be part of the care of teenage women with diabetes, whether they have Type 1 or Type 2 diabetes. It is to be hoped that these teenagers will be attending a teenagers' and young people's clinic at the local diabetes centre, and so counselling should be provided in that context. The issues of good pre-conception glucose control, and folic acid supplementation can also be reinforced if and when a women with diabetes attends the practice for contraceptive advice. Women with diabetes should be advised to present early in pregnancy so that they may be reviewed and referred early.

2. **Early referral of a pregnant women with diabetes to secondary care**

    There needs to be good co-operation between a diabetologist with an interest in pregnancy in diabetes and an obstetrician with a special interest in diabetes, who can run joint clinics to care for women with diabetes throughout their pregnancies. All women with diabetes need to be referred early in pregnancy to such a team for intensive blood glucose control and monitoring throughout pregnancy and delivery. One of the reasons that pregnancy outcome in people with diabetes is not as good as in the population without diabetes is that many pregnancies are unplanned and, as a result, women with diabetes first present late in pregnancy, when they have had poor glycaemic control at the time of conception and first trimester of pregnancy.

3. **Follow up of women diagnosed with gestational diabetes**

Secondary care often used to send women diagnosed as having gestational diabetes for an OGTT around six weeks to three months after delivery to see if their carbohydrate intolerance had returned to normal. They would also attempt to follow these women and invite them back after a year for further testing. Many women do not attend when such appointments are sent and in many areas of the UK the responsibility to follow up women with gestational diabetes has reverted to primary care. Up to 50% of women who have had gestational diabetes will go on to develop Type 2 diabetes, so a yearly follow up with a fasting glucose estimation is good practice.

Pregnancy and women with Type 2 diabetes

Pregnancy care in diabetes used to relate almost exclusively to women with Type 1 diabetes. Type 2 diabetes is now being diagnosed in teenagers in the UK, most of whom are significantly obese. Therefore it is likely that pregnancy in people with Type 2 diabetes who may be treated with diet alone, or diet and metformin, or a combination of diet, metformin and other oral agents will become more common.

Polycystic ovarian syndrome (PCOS)

This syndrome of infertility, irregular periods, hirsutism and polycystic ovaries has been described for many years. A number of women with the syndrome go on to develop Type 2 diabetes. The condition is now thought by many to be caused by insulin resistance in the ovary. Metformin has recently been shown to restore periods and fertility to some women with PCOS, some of whom will have Type 2 diabetes.[5]

Using metformin in this way to restore fertility in women with PCOS, who may also have Type 2 diabetes is not at present a licensed indication for metformin and it is advisable for these women to be monitored in specialist clinics that have the appropriate expertise.

Metformin may have the potential for tetrogenicity and so some authorities suggest that it is advisable to stop it before conception. Good blood glucose control around the time of conception and throughout pregnancy is likely to be important, and so transfering to insulin therapy before conception may be helpful. However, some pregnancies are unplanned and if a women on oral agent therapy presents in early pregnancy, prompt referral to a specialist diabetes/obstetric team and transfer onto insulin will be needed.

Case history

Mrs EG was 35 years old and had had symptoms suggestive of PCOS for eight years, including primary infertility. At the age of 33 she developed Type 2 diabetes and was given metformin 500mg twice daily. Within 18 months she presented with symptoms suggestive of pregnancy, and was urgently referred to a diabetologist with an interest in pregnancy care and an obstetrician with an interest in diabetic pregnancy. Metformin was stopped and she was put on a basal–bolus insulin regime. She remained well-controlled throughout pregnancy and had a healthy baby boy by emergency caesarian section at 38 weeks because of foetal distress. After delivery she was able to transfer off insulin and back onto metformin, and her diabetes remains well-controlled.

Note – in this case history the pregnancy was unplanned. Ideally women should be taken off metformin before conception.

References

1. Kitzmiller JL, Gavin LA, Gin GD *et al.* Preconception care of diabetes. Glycaemic control prevents congenital abnormalities. *JAMA* 1991; **265**: 731–6
2. Scottish   Intercollegiate   Guidelines   Network.   *Management*

   of Diabetes: SIGN guideline 55 Edinburgh: SIGN, Nov 2001 www.sign.ac.uk/guidelines/fulltext/55/index.html (accessed 30 Sept 2004)

3. Jardine-Brown C, Dawson A , Dodds R *et al.* Report of the Pregnancy and Neonatal Care Group. *Diabet Med* 1996; **13**: S43–S53

4. Hanna FWF, Peters JR. Screening for gestational diabetes; past, present and future. *Diabet Med* 2002; **19**: 351–8

5. Lord JM, Flight HK, Norman RJ. Metformin in Polycystic Ovary Syndrome: Systematic review and meta-analysis. *BMJ* 2003; **327**: 951–5

14 ERECTILE DYSFUNCTION (ED)

Erectile dysfunction (ED) is one of the complications of diabetes that used to be rarely mentioned. Treatments for the condition, which causes considerable distress, have become more straightforward in recent years. There is no quality indicator for it in the new GP contract, but it still needs appropriate management.

Background

This is the major sexual problem affecting men with diabetes. It occurs in 30% of all men who have diabetes, rising to 55% in people with diabetes over the age 60.[1] The prevalence and impact of erectile failure in diabetes is probably underestimated because of medical and social taboos. Its aetiology is multifactorial. The main two factors are atheroma causing reduced microvascular blood flow to the penis, and damage to the autonomic nervous system. Psychological factors may also play a part in some people.

Infections, such as balanitis, are common in those with poorly controlled diabetes and can cause malaise, local pain and anxiety, which may all contribute to worsening erectile dysfunction.

Some drugs taken by people with diabetes, such as beta blockers and thiazide diuretics used to treat hypertension, some antidepressants and some anxiolytic agents, are associated with ED. Alcohol, if drunk to excess, may also cause ED.

Now that oral therapy is available to treat ED, men with diabetes are becoming more willing to discuss this microvascular complication.

Trial evidence for the effectiveness of treatments for ED and their use in people with diabetes

Treatment with the agent alprostadil (prostaglandin E1) involves the intra-urethral administration of alprostadil, using a specially designed introducer for self-administration.

Direct injection of vasoactive drugs into the corpus cavernosa of the penis can also be an effective way of producing an erection. The most commonly used drug is alprostadil. The main problem with this form of treatment, as with intra-urethral alprostadil, is overcoming the difficulties and barriers that people may have to injecting into the penis or introducing a substance into the urethra.

Studies have usually been done in general populations of people with ED, which contain numbers of people with diabetes. Few studies have been done in populations with ED and diabetes alone. Satisfaction with treatment rates can approach 75% initially but discontinuation rates approach 50%.[1-2]

The emergence of sildenafil as an oral treatment for erectile dysfunction has been an important breakthrough. It works by suppressing the enzyme phosphodiesterase Type 5 (PDE5), which occurs naturally in the erectile tissue of the penis. PDE5 breaks down intracellular guanosine monophosphate (cGMP), which is produced during arousal and causes the vascular changes that lead to erection of the penis.

Sildenafil is taken an hour or so before intended intercourse. It does not by itself produce arousal, but allows an erection to occur during sexual foreplay. It is available in 25, 50 or 100mg tablets. The stronger doses are needed in people with diabetes and a response rate approaching 60% has been reported.[3]

Two other PDE5 inhibitors have now been released. One is tadalafil and the other vardenafil. More studies are needed to determine the effectiveness of these agents in people with diabetes. It would also be useful to have studies that compare the effectiveness of the three PDE5s with each other, in people with diabetes.

PDE5 inhibitors can interact with nitrate-containing medications to cause hypotension so they should not be used in people with ischaemic heart disease who are taking nitrate therapy.

Vacuum tumescence devices consist of cylinders into which the penis is placed, and from which air is removed creating a vacuum, which then produces an erection. They can be very effective and are free of systemic side effects. Few large-scale studies have been reported so success rates in diabetes are difficult to find.

Statements from guidelines

There are no statements from guidelines.

> **Actions for primary care**
> 1. Be aware of the condition
>   *It is a difficult subject for the person with diabetes and the health care professional to bring up in the consultation. Questions like, 'A number of men with diabetes get problems with getting an erection, is this a problem that is bothering you', can introduce the subject into the consultation in a relatively non-threatening way.*
> 2. Take a brief history
>   *ED due to the microvascular complications of diabetes needs to be distinguished from psychological causes of ED. Table 14.1 lists factors in the history that may distinguish them.*
> 3. Consider changing any therapy that may be making the ED worse
>   *Drugs such as thiazide diuretics, B blockers, antidepressants, and anxiolytic agents may all contribute to ED and should be changed if possible.*

4. Offer treatment options
Psychological causes of ED may improve after discussion and counselling. For ED caused by diabetes, the treatment options of MUSE, Caverjet, vacuum devices and oral PDE5 inhibitors can be discussed. In my experience most opt for a trial of oral therapy. Doses at the upper end of the dose range are usually needed. Diabetes is one of the conditions that allows four oral tablets of a PDE5 inhibitor a month to be prescribed free on the NHS.

Table 14.1 Distinguishing between microvascular and psychological aetiology of ED

	Microvascular	Psychological
Onset	Gradual	Often sudden
Permanence	Intermittent or partial	Total
Nocturnal erections	Never	Sometimes
Psychological symptoms	Absent	Present
Other microvascular complications	Present	Often absent
Erection lost on penetration	No erections	Often happens

Summary points
- ED, which has been described as one of the hidden microvascular complications of diabetes, is now being talked about more openly following the discovery of oral ED therapy.
- Questions about ED need to be raised sensitively at annual review.
- Microvascular causes need to be distinguished from psychological causes.
- Treatment options need to be discussed. Most people opt for a trial of oral PDE5 inhibitor which needs to be given at the upper end of its dose range.

References

1. Lakin MM, Montague DK, Vanderbrig Medendorp S *et al.* Intracavernous injection therapy: analysis of results and complications. *J Urol* 1990; **143:** 1138–41

2. Spollett GR. Assessment and management of erectile dysfunction in men with diabetes. *Diabetes Educator* 1999; **25:** 65–73

3. Rendell MS, Rajfer J, Wicker P *et al* for the Sildenafil Diabetes Study Group. Sildenafil for treatment of erectile dysfunction in men with diabetes: a randomised controlled study. *JAMA* 1999; **281:** 421–6

ACUTE COMPLICATIONS

The acute complications of diabetes do not directly figure in the quality and outcomes framework. However, they are such an important part of diabetes care that they need to be discussed.

Hypoglycaemia

Background

Hypoglycaemia is a common symptom of treatment with insulin and some sulphonylureas.

Incidence rates for severe hypoglycaemia, (defined as needing help from health care personnel) in a Scottish community survey were 11.5 and 11.8 events per 100 patient years in Type 1 and Type 2 diabetes treated with insulin. In the study period, 7.1% of people with Type 1 diabetes, 7.3% of people with Type 2 diabetes treated with insulin, and 0.8% of people treated with a sulphonylurea had a severe hypoglycaemic episode. Age, duration of diabetes and socioeconomic status, were identified as risk factors for severe hypoglycaemia.[1]

Symptoms

They are classified into two groups, autonomic and neuroglycopenic.

Autonomic symptoms:
- sweating
- pounding heart
- shakiness or tremor
- hunger.

These are due to activation of the sympathetic or parasympathetic nervous system.

Neuroglycopenic symptoms:
- confusion
- drowsiness

- difficulty with speech
- lack of co-ordination
- double vision
- atypical behaviour, e.g. aggression.

These symptoms are due to the effects of glucose deprivation on the brain and may develop at different levels of low blood glucose in different people. However, most people will get symptoms when glucose levels drop to below 3 mmol/l.

Hypoglycaemic unawareness is when an individual loses the early warning signs of impending hypoglycaemia and goes from feeling well, to profound symptomatic hypoglycaemia without symptomatic warning and therefore is unable to take any action to alleviate the problem. People who have hypoglycaemic unawareness may have significant problems with driving.

Unawareness increases with duration of diabetes, in situations of repeated hypoglycaemia, where there is autonomic neuropathy and in situations of intensive glycaemic control. Hypoglycaemia should be confirmed by a finger prick blood glucose test if possible. The management of hypoglycaemia depends on the level of consciousness and co-operation of the patient.

If the person is conscious and co-operative:
- provide a sugary drink, e.g. a glass of milk with four spoons of sugar in it, or three or four glucose sweets
- follow this with a substantial snack or meal high in carbohydrate
- check blood glucose levels to ensure that they have returned to normal.

If the person is conscious but unco-operative:
- use dextrose gel (Hypostop). Insert gel into the mouth, using around a third of the bottle, massage gently around the cheeks to aid absorption of the gel through the buccal mucosa.
- repeat the steps above as for co-operative state.

If the person is unconscious:

- give glucagon injection subcutaneou tramuscular (IM)
- place the person in the recovery positi return of consciousness which usually to 20 minutes.

If glucagon doesn't render the person conscious:

- Contact ambulance. Paramedics or medical personnel can then give an intravenous injection (IV) of glucose, usually in the form of 20ml of 25% or 50% glucose solution given into a large vein through a wide-bore needle.

Great caution is needed with venous access as concentrated glucose solutions can damage tissue if they leak out of a vein, so care must be given to ensure that this does not occur.

Sulphonylurea-induced hypoglycaemia

This risk mainly occurs with the long acting sulphonylureas, like chlorpropramide and glibenclamide. Hypoglycaemia may recur again after an initial episode has been successfully treated, so people with long-acting sulphonylurea-induced hypoglycaemia should be admitted to hospital where they can be monitored closely and given a dextrose drip. Hypoglycaemia may cause elderly people to fall, and so long-acting sulphonylureas should not be used in older people.

Hyperglycaemic states

Introduction

There are two hyperglycaemic conditions both of which are serious and which are associated with a significant risk of mortality. One is diabetic ketoacidosis (DKA); the other is hyperosmolar non-ketotic coma (HONK).

In DKA the main biochemical abnormalities are raised blood glucose levels, raised ketone levels and acidosis. It occurs in situations of insulin deficiency found in Type 1 diabetes.

In HONK the glucose levels are usually extremely elevated, there is dehydration but no ketosis. The absence of ketosis may be because of residual endogenous insulin production in Type 2 diabetes, because hyperosmolality suppresses lipolysis or because counter-regulatory hormone responses are less well-developed.

Table 15.1   Possible causes of DKA and HONK

DKA	HONK
Infection	Infection
Omission of insulin injection	Undiagnosed Type 2 diabetes
Inadequate insulin injection	CVA
Previously undiagnosed Type 1 diabetes	Myocardial infarction
	Acute pancreatitis

Signs and symptoms

In DKA the symptoms are: thirst, polyuria, weight loss, weakness, nausea, leg cramps, drowsiness and eventually coma. Abdominal pain may occur. Signs include: dehydration, hypotension, tachycardia, hyperventilation and a sweet smell on the breath.

In HONK the symptoms are similar minus the ones associated with ketosis.

Treatment

People with hyperglycaemic states need to be admitted for close monitoring, IV rehydration, potassium supplementation as necessary, and IV insulin infusion.

Actions for primary care

1. Ensure that people with diabetes are educated in looking after themselves when they get illness or infection observing the 'sick day rules' (see Box 15.1).
2. Ensure that the level of dehydration and blood glucose levels are monitored during illness.
3. Admit, if the person's clinical condition deteriorates.

Box 15.1 Sick day rules for people with diabetes

- Minor illness (e.g. colds and 'flu) may cause blood glucose levels to rise temporarily. It is therefore important that they monitor their levels more frequently while they are unwell.
- People with diabetes should continue to take their medications for diabetes (tablets and/or insulin).
- Drink extra fluids.
- Vomiting and diarrhoea may result in the loss of a high volume of fluid. Recommend drinking extra fluids. Sips of glucose-containing drinks are safe and useful in these circumstances.
- It is safe to take paracetamol to reduce high temperatures, and for headache and sore throat symptoms.
- It is safe to take sugar-free cough remedies.
- If the person is not hungry, they can substitute solid meals with liquids or light diet (e.g. soups, milk, glucose drinks or ice cream).
- If vomiting or illness persists, people with diabetes will need to contact their doctor for further advice.

References

1. Leese G, Wang J, Broomhall J *et al*. Frequency of severe hypoglycaemia requiring emergency treatment in Type 1 and Type 2 diabetes. *Diabetes Care* **26**: 1176–80

People on diet or diet and tablets

Those treated with diet alone, or on diet and oral medications can undertake most occupations as the risk of hypoglycaemia is small.

Some of the employment restrictions encountered in the UK may have been established by individual companies or industries rather than by legislation. Diabetes UK campaigns for individual assessment of risk in employment, taking into account the type and method of diabetes treatment, rather than blanket bans.

Actions for primary care

Diabetes UK has a wealth of information and accounts of people with diabetes campaigning for individual assessment and being able to successfully continue in employment. Anyone with employment concerns should be encouraged to contact Diabetes UK for assistance.

Travel

People with diabetes should experience few problems with long-distance travel providing they have planned in advance. It is important to obtain travel insurance declaring diabetes in order to obtain adequate cover.

Insulin and accessories should be carried in hand luggage. It will freeze and be rendered ineffective if it is kept in luggage that goes in the cargo hold of an aircraft. In these times of high security, a written statement from a health care professional confirming diabetes and the need to carry insulin, accessories and needles is helpful.

Insulin absorption may be increased in hot climates, and there is a risk of damage to insensitive feet from walking on hot sand. An extended day that occurs during a long westward airplane flight may require an additional dose of short-acting insulin.

> **Actions for primary care**
> Provide helpful advice and support for people with diabetes who are contemplating travel. Get specialist advice, perhaps from Diabetes UK, if there are particular issues around the need for an extra injection of short-acting insulin.

Alcohol

Alcohol lowers blood glucose levels, so it is important not to drink on an empty stomach. Alcohol can be taken in moderation by people who have diabetes. The maximum recommendations are for three units per day for men and two units per day for women.

Alcohol abuse is dangerous in people with diabetes because hypoglycaemia can pass undetected in inebriated people. There is some evidence that low, regular alcohol intake e.g. one or two glasses of wine per day may reduce the risk of cardiovascular complications.

> **Actions for primary care**
> Discuss alcohol intake as part of initial and on-going education in people with diabetes.